A Quick Start Guide to Methadone Maintenance Counseling

A QUICK START GUIDE TO METHADONE MAINTENANCE COUNSELING

by
Abraham H. Kou, LPC, CAADC

foreword by
Karen Y. Mechanic, MD

Copyright © 2018 by Abraham H. Kou

All rights reserved. No part of this publication may be reproduced, distributed, or transmitted in any form or by any means, including photocopying, recording, or other electronic or mechanical methods, without the prior written permission of the publisher, except in the case of brief quotations embodied in critical reviews and certain other noncommercial uses permitted by copyright law.

Edited by:
Samantha Wright

Cover design by:
oliviaprodesign

SUBOXONE® and SUBUTEX® are registered trademarks of Indivior UK Limited.

VIVITROL® is a registered trademark of Alkermes, Inc.

NARCAN® is a registered trademark of ADAPT Pharma Operations Limited.

PERCOCET® is a registered trademark of Endo Pharmaceuticals Inc.

KLONOPIN® is a registered trademark of Genentech Inc.

XANAX® is a registered trademark of Pharmacy and Upjohn Company LLC.

CATAPRES® is a registered trademark of Boehringer Ingelheim Pharmaceuticals Inc.

DOLOPHINE® is a registered trademark of Roxane Laboratories Inc.

For Lorrain and Ellie

Contributors

Dennis J. Hand, PhD, Assistant Professor, Departments of Obstetrics & Gynecology and Psychiatry & Human Behavior, Thomas Jefferson University

Emily Loscalzo, PsyD, Assistant Professor, Department of Psychiatry & Human Behavior, Thomas Jefferson University

Karen Y. Mechanic, MD, Associate Clinical Professor, Department of Psychiatry & Human Behavior, Thomas Jefferson University

Meghan Morley, LPC, Certified Personal Trainer, Certified Group Fitness Instructor, Lead Patient Navigator, Department of Psychiatry & Human Behavior, Thomas Jefferson University

Foreword
Karen Y. Mechanic, MD

Methadone has been an approved medical treatment for opioid use disorder in the United States since 1972 (National Archives and Records Administration, 1972).

While there are other forms of treatment available for people who struggle with opioid addiction, methadone maintenance has been proven to be more effective than many treatments (Ball & Ross, 2012). Methadone is not a panacea; there are other alternatives such as buprenorphine, naltrexone, and non-medication options. Successful methadone patients can, however, have all the benefits and pleasures in life anyone could ask for because they work, have stable housing, enjoy meaningful relationships, complete their education, and attend to their medical needs.

This book results from many conversations among a group of dedicated addiction treatment professionals. We are inspired by our work—constantly seeking to help each other understand how to assist those who have sought our expertise. These folks are patients but also family members, other medical professionals and those who simply want to understand more about the opioid crisis.

This manual is a must read for anyone curious about opioid addiction. We offer a window into its world, as it is a primer written by professionals taught by education and experience. They have given their time and attention to create this handbook aiming to educate by providing evidence and facts about methadone maintenance treatment.

The chapters cover topics germane to the medication (pharmacologic treatment) and the practice of methadone counseling. These experts in treatment have written about pharmacology, pregnancy, exercise, and diet, as well as spirituality. The glossary and images in this book are also helpful and educational.

We respect our patients, learn from them, and hope you will also.

Karen Y. Mechanic, MD

Contents

Introduction 2

1: The Basics of Methadone Maintenance 5
    Why MMT Works 6
    How Does Methadone Work? 7
    What Is the Difference Between Methadone and Buprenorphine? 8
    Increases, Split-Dosing, and Stabilization 9
    Post-Stabilization: Take-Home Dosages and Guest Dosing 10
    Looking Further: Possible Methadone Detoxification 11
    Even Further: Naltrexone for Relapse Prevention After MMT 12
    How Mental Health Professionals Fit into MMT 13
    Summary 15

2: Phases of Treatment 16
    From Induction to Rehabilitation: Phases 1 to 3 17
    Phase 4: A Decision Point 17
    Phase 4C: Maintaining Gains from Treatment 19
    Summary 20

3: Maternal Opioid Addiction 22
    Why Opioid Agonists? 22

    Dosing Considerations in Pregnancy 23

    Risks and Side-Effects 23

    Postpartum Considerations 26

    Developmental Effects of Prenatal Opioid Exposure 26

    Summary 27

4: Risks Associated with MMT 28

    General Side Effects 28

    Risk of Overdose 32

    Withdrawal 33

    Driving 34

    Methadone Diversion 34

    Summary 38

5: Harm Reduction 39

    MMT and Harm Reduction 39

    Overdose Education and Response 40

    Provision of Medical and Psychiatric Services 42

    Referrals to Appropriate Levels of Care 43

    Summary 43

6: Trauma and Chemical Dependency 45

    Evidence-Based Treatments for PTSD 46

    Herman's Stages of Trauma Recovery 47

    Prolonged Exposure Therapy (PE) 49

Cognitive Processing Therapy (CPT) 51

Eye Movement Desensitization and Reprocessing Therapy (EMDR) . 52

Summary 53

7: Motivational Interviewing 54

The Stages of Change 54

What is Motivational Interviewing (MI)? 55

Assessing Readiness to Change 56

Exploring Client Change with O.A.R.S. 57

"Change Talk" Versus "Sustain Talk" 58

Summary 59

8: Involving Loved Ones in Treatment 60

Family of Origin Considerations for Treating Chemical Dependency 60

The Role of Family Sessions in Treatment 61

Triangulation and Why It Matters 62

Supporting the Family Through the Immediate Community 63

Summary 64

9: Support 65

An Overview of Peer Support 65

Support from Inside the Treatment Setting 66

Community Support 67

Summary 70

10: Spirituality	71
"A Spiritual Awakening"	72
Bridging Spirituality with Mental Health Counseling	72
Spirituality and Self-Help Groups	73
Support from Religious Communities	73
Summary	74
11: Nutrition and Exercise	75
Nutrition	76
Exercise	81
Summary	83
Common Myths and Facts About MMT	84
Useful Websites	86
Useful Books	95
Glossary	97
References	107

Introduction

People are hurting. Whether they are the child that came home after a long trip to find that their parents had packed their bags and abandoned them, or perhaps the loyal spouse of twenty years that recently lost their partner, they are hurting on the inside.

Our society tries to treat physical pain. We can see the wounds inflicted, and with the help of Western medicine prescribe the proper medication.

Emotional pain can be harder to grasp because we cannot see it. Although modern psychotherapy has come a long way since classical Freudian psychoanalysis, it is still a budding art and science. A certain sense of guilt and shame can emerge from having a condition we do not fully understand how to treat into complete remission. This can be frustrating and scary for those that suffer, and for the people around them.

With the release of the U.S. Surgeon General's report in 2017, we continue to change how we understand addiction. Modern neurobiology has told us there is confidence in the notion that addiction is a disease of the brain. Pronounced members of the medical field, such as National Institute on Drug Abuse (NIDA) director Nora Volkow, MD, are advocating this view; there is science supporting there are meaningful biological changes that occur from chronic substance misuse and process addictions.

Treatment is readily available, and there are many roads to recovery from problems caused by substance use. Evidence-based therapeutic modalities and medication-assisted treatments provide hope for those suffering.

There is no other medical condition that affects so many aspects of a person's life: biological, psychological, social, spiritual - well, every facet of human experience. Our clients need a team of supporters, like yourself, to reach a point of wellness.

To you, the reader: thank you for taking your time to continually refine your practice and learn more about those we serve. This is not meant to be an infallible and indisputable reference for working with methadone maintenance treatment (MMT). Also, this guide is not a commentary on MMT's regulation and how it may impact clients, which differs state-by-state, and country-to-country.

Given the nuanced nature of methadone maintenance, it is the hope that this book will be utilized for future clinicians who may not have prior experience with MMT and are hoping to be a part of the participants' healing process.

1: The Basics of Methadone Maintenance

"Physicians today are providing the leadership to help end the nation's opioid-related overdose and death epidemic. As medical professionals, we go where the evidence leads us."
– Patrice A. Harris, MD, MA

Methadone maintenance treatment (MMT) is an evidenced-based medication-assisted treatment used for the corrective treatment of the DSM-5 diagnostic criteria for opioid use disorder (American Psychiatric Association, 2013). It relies on methadone, which is a synthetic opioid medication that activates μ-opioid receptors in the brain. Methadone comes in liquid, pills, and wafers. MMT has been around in the world since the 1950s (WHO, 2009).

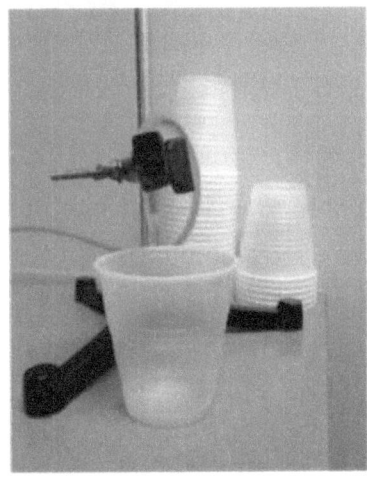

Figure 1. Liquid methadone being prepared to dispense to clients.

Why MMT Works

The theory behind MMT consists of treating opioid dependency by giving a medically-monitored medication that will help a client wean cravings and physical withdrawal associated with illicit opioids. While they receive methadone, it is the anticipation that they will also thrive from the additional medical and psychotherapy services offered in the treatment environment.

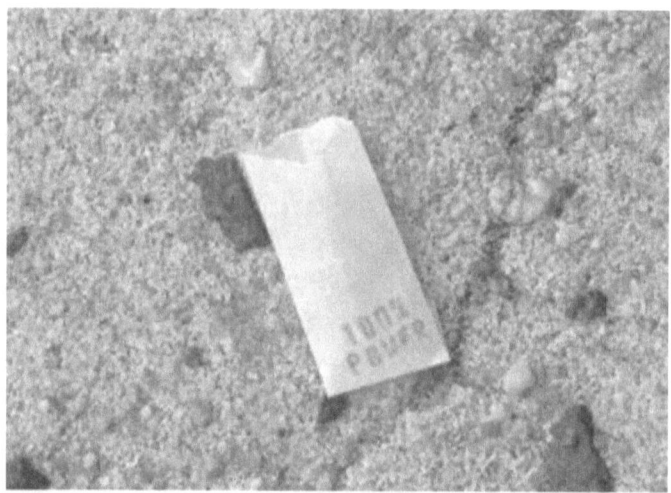

Figure 2. A blue glassine bag of *China White* heroin littering a street in Philadelphia, PA.

The pure nature of the prescribed methadone is much safer compared to street heroin that is often intermixed with things like sugars, starch, powdered milk, quinine, and other chemicals resulting from crude processing (NIDA, 2018b). Within these concoctions, an increase of adding fentanyl has also been leading to more opioid-related deaths (Pichini, Solimini, Berretta, Pacifici, & Busardò, 2017).

With repeated use of such illicit opioids being so dangerous, MMT can be a form of treatment that has the potential of preserving a client's life. This is given that substance addiction is a chronic medical condition that has a probability for relapse (McLellan, Lewis, O'brien, & Kleber, 2000). Subsequently, participants taking prescribed methadone are less likely to resume use of these illicit opioids and severely injure themselves or die.

To this point, there has been research that is consistent in suggesting that it provides decreased use of illicit opioid use and better treatment retention compared to non-opioid replacement programs (Ball & Ross, 2012; Connock et al., 2007; Marsch, 1998; Mattick, Breen, Kimber, & Davoli, 2009). In addition, MMT has demonstrated that it can reduce rates of mortality, additional contact with the criminal justice system, and rates of hepatitis C infection (Dolan et al., 2005).

How Does Methadone Work?

Methadone is a full opioid agonist that activates μ-opioid receptors in the brain. These receptors are proteins that are located on the surface of nerve cells that communicate with one another through chemical messengers or neurotransmitters. When a client takes their prescribed dosage, it can provide 24-36 hours (with a range of 13-56 hours) of relief from withdrawal symptoms and cravings (Kleber, 2008). A good way to think of how these receptor sites are satiated is imagining locks (receptors) and keys (agonists) within your brain.

Opioid drugs, like methadone, mimic similar naturally-occurring molecules in the brain that help control pain, immune response, and other bodily functions. Within addiction, opioids play a central role in drug reward, broadly in: altered reward processing, disruption in emotional responses, and poor decision-making (Lutz & Kieffer, 2013).

What Is the Difference Between Methadone and Buprenorphine?

The difference between methadone and popular forms of buprenorphine treatments (i.e., Suboxone® and Subutex®) is that methadone completely fills this opioid receptor site and does not have a ceiling effect. Conversely, buprenorphine medications are considered partial agonists that fill up some of these receptor sites rather than all.

A ceiling effect is the level that a medication stops becoming incrementally effective when increasing its dosage. In other words, the more methadone a client takes, the higher the probability that cravings for opioids are reduced, withdrawal symptoms are alleviated, and euphoria from opioids is blocked.

Most clients are stabilized around 80 mg to 120 mg of methadone daily (Joseph, Stancliff, & Langrod, 2000; Mallinckrodt Pharmaceuticals Inc., 2008; Vocci, Acri, & Elkashef, 2005). However, a participant may be assessed by a physician to receive more medication than this to stop illicit opioid use. In contrast, the benefits associated with higher amounts of buprenorphine are capped at a maintenance dosage of 16 mg (Indivior Inc., 2018).

Although methadone and buprenorphine are medications that activate these opioid receptor sites, one may be better tailored than another during a client's course of treatment. As such, a comprehensive evaluation by an addiction medicine physician is necessary for determining the most appropriate medication and its therapeutic dosage for helping a client treat their opioid dependency.

With this in mind, each client that passes through our doors is unique. There might be individuals who may require different dosages of methadone that could be higher, lower, or even split across two to three distinct amounts at varying times of the day (split-dosing); perhaps even a different type of medication-assisted treatment altogether.

Increases, Split-Dosing, and Stabilization

"I need an increase" is a phrase that all staff members hear often.

Constant re-evaluation of cases is important, given that people can have substantially different medical and psychosocial histories. A participant may request assistance in coordinating an assessment for an increase of medication if their dosage does not feel right. This is often indicated by a lack of suppression in cravings and withdrawal symptoms, plus continued use of illicit opioids.

As such, these increases can be instrumental in helping a client wean off these additional opioids they may be using. Literature shows that adding higher and higher dosages of methadone is often correlated with a greater suppression of illicit opioid use (Strain, Stitzer, Liebson, & Bigelow, 1993). Such greater dosages can sometimes be attributed to underlying psychopathology, persistent opiate use, or symptoms of incomplete coverage by methadone (Maremmani, Pacini, Lubrano, & Lovrecic, 2003).

To reiterate, if a client feels as though their dosage does not feel right, they need to be assessed for a higher dosage of medication by medical and nursing personnel. When a dosage does not "hold" a client, it is important to look at the entire clinical picture. To this, Baxter et al. (2013) recommend that we examine several dimensions with our interdisciplinary team: continued illicit opioid use, medical or psychiatric conditions, and rapid metabolization.

Methadone is metabolized in the liver. Variations in enzyme activity can often account for differences in methadone metabolism between patients (Leavitt, Shinderman, Maxwell, Eap, & Paris, 2013). Blood work reporting a methadone peak and trough through serum or plasma can be ordered at the discretion of the medical director to help inform whether a participant may need a split-dosage of methadone for combating withdrawal later in the day. A client could be a rapid metabolizer who would feel less discomfort receiving one dosage in the morning, as well as one much later. There are country and state regulation considerations for split-dosing, plus diversion concerns addressed later in Chapter 4.

Following additional laboratory testing, consultation with outside specialists, such as a cardiologist, can be paramount in addressing potentially unresolved issues within methadone stabilization. As we will look at in Chapter 2, this entire stabilization period is predominantly focused on reaching an optimal dosage of methadone, minimizing illicit drug use, and addressing any acute medical difficulties.

Post-Stabilization: Take-Home Dosages and Guest Dosing

Depending on the country, state, and facility regulations with MMT, a client has the potential to earn take-home dosages. Such doses are typically earned through testing negative for illicit substances and demonstrating good standing with the treatment environment. Methadone dosages issued to the client are intended to minimize their contact with their clinic and promote autonomy.

If a participant does not have take-home privileges and needs to travel, careful guest dosing coordination may be organized by the treatment provider. This is where your clinic generates a guest dosing request to be received by the clinic at the participant's final destination.

Before they may be sent, it is recommended that they are in good standing with the clinic, at a stable dosage of methadone, and have medical plus psychiatric stability.

Arrangements are often made one to two weeks before the client travels, by contacting the receiving clinic and reviewing their guest dosing protocol, which will also include any payment or required identification that a participant will bring.

Typically, several components are confidentially faxed, mailed, or emailed prior to the client's arrival: a release of information, basic demographic information, a list of current medications, and a last dose confirmation of methadone. It can be good practice to issue a copy of this last dose confirmation to the client, as well as provide the address of the receiving clinic with dispensing hours to the traveling participant.

Possible considerations for those traveling internationally may be located at https://indro-online.de/en/methadone-worldwide-travel-guide/.

Looking Further: Possible Methadone Detoxification

Even from the beginning of treatment, it is important to ask about a client's long-term goals surrounding their methadone dosage. A participant will either maintain taking a dosage of methadone for medical purposes, or they may consider tapering.

On-going counseling and consultation from an interdisciplinary team will help a person consider whether they have reached a stable place in their rehabilitation to reduce their dosage. It may vary where you are working at, but this is commonly evidenced by:

- Having a consistent home and work life.
- Identifying and engaging in drug-free recreational activities.
- Immersing in a sober social support network.
- Managing potential medical and psychiatric concerns.

Concurrent coordination of care with a physician is paramount in determining a detoxification plan with the participant. A prescription of naltrexone may be a part of relapse prevention following methadone detoxification.

Even Further: Naltrexone for Relapse Prevention After MMT

Naltrexone is another form of medication-assisted treatment that is used to treat opioid dependency. It is considered an opioid antagonist, which means that it blocks opioid receptor sites, so an individual does not experience euphoria from using opioids (Kosten & George, 2002). As such, a potential participant would need to wean off all opioids and not be experiencing withdrawal symptoms before trying this treatment modality.

Unlike methadone and buprenorphine, it does not stop drug cravings and is recommended for those in an early stage of opioid addiction. Naltrexone is also prescribed to treat alcohol dependency (SAMHSA, 2009). It comes in pill form, as well as an extended-release injectable form called Vivitrol® (CSAT, 2009).

As with any prescription medication, there are potential side effects and risks associated with a fatal overdose if an individual resumes use of substances. It is necessary to consult with a prescribing physician regarding the risks of receiving this form of treatment.

How Mental Health Professionals Fit into MMT

Given the complex nature of the disease of addiction, the role of a counselor is often multifaceted. Agencies can differ in their expectations of duties based on staffing needs. Also, the delineations between standards within different licenses can also have an impact (e.g., LFMT, LPC, LSW, LCSW).

Methadone counselors may perform several of these duties, if not more:

Individual counseling
- Screening and assessment for substance use and mental health challenges.
- Treatment planning that integrates relapse prevention strategies, building coping skills, and developing a sober social support network.
- Administering psychoeducation on the phases of methadone maintenance, the disease of addiction, and principles of harm reduction.
- Providing Motivational Interviewing to reconcile ambivalence towards the potential on-going substance use and adherence to treatment.
- Making recommendations for, or helping to provide adjunctive therapies: art, equine, horticultural, massage, music, recreation, social enrichment, etc.

Group counseling
- Facilitating core interpersonal process groups, as well as specialty topic groups pertinent to methadone-maintained clients.

Couple's and family counseling
- Performing psychoeducation on the treatment goals and phases of methadone maintenance.
- Introducing stigma management of methadone-maintained status, and addressing concerns that loved ones have with the treatment modality.

Comprehensive case management
- Connecting participants with community resources: meals in the area, shelter, support groups, transportation, additional mental health providers, etc.
- Designing continuing support plans, which may include: recommendations for higher levels of care, transitioning to other types of medication-assisted treatments, recovery/halfway housing, and/or outpatient mental health care.

Coordination of care with medical and nursing staff
- Corresponding with outside physicians involved in client care, which could include discussion of methadone dosage.
- Helping to organize guest dosing at receiving clinic if a participant is interested in travel.

Supervision of interns or other clinical staff members

Summary

Methadone maintenance is an evidence-based type of medication-assisted treatment that has provided hope and stability to those in recovery. Along with preserving life, methadone coupled with psychotherapy allows an individual to rehabilitate without the biological cravings associated with illicit opioids.

It has several phases of treatment and notable differences compared to buprenorphine or naltrexone-based treatments. These options are definitely important to explore with a potential client while they are being thoroughly assessed for a methadone maintenance program.

Once on-boarded and matched with a counselor, a mental health provider may wear any number of different hats while working with participants. This may include (and is not limited to) individual counseling, group counseling, couples' and family counseling, comprehensive case management, and supervision. While providing these services, coordinating care with medical providers, such as physicians and nurses, is paramount.

2: Phases of Treatment

Induction into treatment begins with informed consent, participant and family education, and the first dosage of methadone. This entry into treatment often extends into the first two weeks and is a period of documented assessment and monitoring (Baxter et al., 2013).

While a client is getting to know the ropes of a treatment program and navigate changes happening in their bodies and brains, let them know what is to come in the next few days and weeks. Adding attention to their overall adjustment and addressing any concerns or questions can have a strong influence on the direction of treatment. With that being said, having a blueprint to guide and inform treatment is an integral part of MMT.

The Phases of Treatment Model (Moolchan & Hoffman, 1994) offers a means of structuring methadone maintenance and provides guidelines for the treatment process.

Below, there is an illustration and summary of each phase:

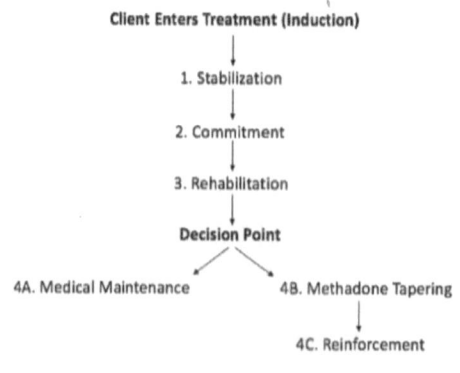

Figure 3. The Phases of Treatment Model (Moolchan & Hoffman, 1994).

From Induction to Rehabilitation: Phases 1 to 3

The first three phases of treatment are focused on bringing someone into care, stabilizing their dosage while minimizing illicit opioid use, offering treatment for medical and psychiatric issues, and integrating community support. Phases 1 to 3 are outlined below:

1. **Stabilization:** coordinating care with medical and nursing staff to reach an optimal dosage of methadone, minimizing illicit drug use, and addressing any acute medical difficulties. An assessment tool like the Clinical Opiate Withdrawal Scale (COWS) developed by Wesson and Ling (2003) may be employed to help determine adjustments with medication.
2. **Commitment:** the focus is on instilling hope in the client for a better lifestyle. Motivational Interviewing can help resolve ambivalence in taking steps towards holistic wellness (see Chapter 7).
3. **Rehabilitation:** begin working and participating in family and community life. Clients start demonstrating a different lifestyle outside of drug subculture.

Phase 4: A Decision Point

According to the Phases Model, a client successfully participating in rehabilitation will then decide on whether to begin methadone tapering or continue with indefinite medical maintenance. In theory, a client enjoying holistic stability may think about the prospect of tapering, which houses unique concerns in relapse prevention.

Within this decision point, Moolchan & Hoffman (1994) state that clients have two choices: indefinite medical maintenance or downward titration of their dosage.

4A. **Medical maintenance:** this is a recommended option for clients that may become medically compromised from a detox. An additional consideration involves the risk of potential resumed use of illicit substances while detoxing, and how this may significantly affect a client's well-being.

In this phase, a participant might earn multiple take-home dosages depending on their clinic's rules and regulations, plus minimize their contact with the facility.

4B. **Methadone tapering:** this consists of a gradual reduction of methadone dosage to medication-free status with the ideal of no resumed use of illicit substances during and after the detoxification. Within this phase, it is crucial to utilize sober social support and relapse prevention skills practiced during the "Rehabilitation" stage.

The mental health professional must help the participant explore whether they have reached a point of stability with their maintenance dosage of methadone and holistic wellness before gradually tapering. Clinically, it can be worthwhile to collaboratively explore the success of managing pre-existing medical and psychiatric issues and current life circumstances before detoxification is considered. As mentioned in Chapter 1, such circumstances for a taper may include a regular work routine, improvement of family life, identification of drug-free recreational activities, and immersion in a sober social support network.

If a participant begins a taper, it is especially important to have regular contact with them and further integrate sober social support. In fact, qualitative research shows us that having a trusted health care provider monitor the detox, as well as receiving support from family members or peers, can make a significant difference (Frank et al., 2016).

Research is limited in what predictive factors are linked to a lack of resumed use during and following methadone detoxification. Cushman (1974) suggested that some of these elements may include: a slower speed with tapering, full-time employment, the positive motivation for detoxification, and reintegration into an environment that is not conducive towards continued drug use. Additional review of existing literature also indicates that successful tapering is often paired with gradual dose reductions with periods of stabilization before reinitiating the detox (Nosyk et al., 2012).

Close coordination with the prescribing physician and nursing staff is key for developing and carefully evaluating a detoxification plan that considers the unique medical and psychosocial histories of a client. Again, sometimes a participant and a provider may decide that a longer or indefinite period of maintenance may be what is best for the overall quality of life for an individual. This does not equate failure in treatment.

Phase 4C: Maintaining Gains from Treatment

After a client's last dosage of methadone, it is important to celebrate this part of their journey. Additionally, on-going continuing support planning is critical in maintaining the progress a participant has made.

4C. **Reinforcement:** During this phase, a client is considered medication-free following their last dosage of methadone. In such a time period, coping and relapse prevention skills learned in counseling are necessary to maintain abstinence from illicit substances. Involvement in an on-going sober social support network (12-step group, support group, and/or religious institution) can also be valuable.

The Phases of Treatment Model offers a means of providing a framework to guide treatment for both clinicians and clients, alike. Ideally, a client undergoing MMT stabilizes with their methadone dosage, minimizes their substance use, makes changes within their lifestyle, and learns how deal with high-risk situations for potential resumed use. They may engage in a methadone detox once their quality of life and health has improved substantially.

Of course, prior to helping a client make their own decisions surrounding any major adjustments to their medication, it is always important to explore both the advantages and disadvantages associated with this decision. Ultimately, respecting the autonomy of a client to make their own decisions and learn from possible mistakes is a critical value to exercise in the counseling process.

Summary

Methadone maintenance has several phases of treatment important for both the provider and the consumer to understand thoroughly. The moment that a client is brought into our program, it is crucial to provide informed consent and information surrounding the treatment model before the first dose is administered.

Following this, a client works towards stabilizing their dosage beginning with a thorough assessment by medical and nursing personnel at a program. After stabilization is achieved, which is typically established through a lack of physical withdrawal symptoms and cravings for illicit opioids, groundwork can be laid on fully committing to the treatment model.

Rehabilitation through improvement of all aspects of the individual, such as physical health, mental well-being, home and work stability, and learning plus practicing relapse prevention skills can be aspects of this phase.

Typically, after around two years of methadone maintenance, a comprehensive and on-going assessment by both the treatment team and the client is completed to determine whether methadone tapering or continued medical maintenance is imperative to maintaining sobriety.

3: Maternal Opioid Addiction
Dennis J. Hand, PhD

Maintenance with methadone or buprenorphine combined with comprehensive counseling and behavioral health care is the recommended standard care for pregnant women with opioid use disorder by the American College of Obstetricians & Gynecologists (ACOG Committee on Health Care for Underserved Women, 2012) and the American Society of Addiction Medicine (Kampman & Jarvis, 2015). Medication-assisted withdrawal is not recommended for pregnant women with opioid use disorder due to high rates of relapse to illicit opioid use (Terplan et al., 2018).

Why Opioid Agonists?

Opioid agonists prevent withdrawal and cravings, in turn reducing the use of illicitly-obtained opioids. Reducing such use lessens risks of infections, such as Hepatitis B and C, HIV, and other infections that could be transmitted to the fetus or otherwise jeopardize the pregnancy. Opioid agonist maintenance also reduces cycling between abstinence and use due to fluctuations in street drug quality and availability and a person's own attempts to abstain. Although opioid detoxification itself does not appear to produce significant danger to the fetus, high rates of relapse to opioid use following detoxification make it an unappealing alternative (Terplan et al., 2018).

Generally, opioid agonists used for medication-assisted treatment are safe for both maternal and infant health. Rates of preterm birth tend to be higher and birth weights tend to be lower in this population compared to non-exposed pregnancies. These effects are less likely to result from opioid agonist maintenance and are more concretely associated with poor maternal nutrition, and co-occurring use of other substances, particularly tobacco products.

Up to 95% of pregnant women with opioid use disorder also use tobacco products (Akerman et al., 2015). Tobacco use during pregnancy is causally related to pregnancy complications like intrauterine growth restriction, preterm birth and birth defects like cleft lip and cleft palate (Cnattingius, 2004). It is imperative that tobacco product use is addressed during treatment for opioid use disorder during pregnancy.

Dosing Considerations in Pregnancy

Split-dosing of agonists is commonly necessary during pregnancy due to increased metabolism. In the postpartum period, the agonist dose should be reduced gradually to avoid oversedation while also preventing withdrawal and cravings from returning.

Risks and Side-Effects

Newborns exposed to opioids, including methadone and buprenorphine, during gestation may experience withdrawal symptoms shortly after birth, often called Neonatal Abstinence Syndrome (NAS). Opioid withdrawal signs in newborns are similar to those in adults, including vomiting, diarrhea, sweating, and tremors in extremities. Rarely, newborns can have seizures during withdrawal from opioids. In most hospitals, a newborn's withdrawal is assessed for 3-5 days, with observer-rated scales conducted every 3-6 hours. Newborns' withdrawal symptoms peak between 24-72 hours after birth (Gaalema et al., 2012). Approximately 50% of opioid-exposed newborns will experience withdrawal that is severe enough to require a pharmacological intervention.

It is important to remember that NAS is a temporary and manageable condition. Many hospitals have protocols for providing comfort care to opioid-exposed newborns. Swaddling, skin-to-skin contact, breastfeeding, and maintaining a low light and quiet environment can help reduce newborn withdrawal symptoms (Velez & Jansson, 2008). If the newborn's withdrawal symptoms become severe, the newborn may be administered opioid agonists, such as morphine, methadone, or buprenorphine. A physician will gradually increase the amount of opioid given until withdrawal symptoms are stabilized, and then gradually reduce the dose over the course of several days.

NAS is a chief concern of pregnant women with opioid use disorder and it has received significant publicity as a costly result of the opioid epidemic, with annual costs in the United States eclipsing $1.5 billion (Patrick et al., 2012). NAS can also be a source of guilt and shame for the mother, both self-imposed and imposed by others. Understanding what influences NAS and considering possible trade-offs for treatment decisions is critical.

What does not affect NAS?
A mother's dose of methadone or buprenorphine is not associated with the risk of her newborn requiring opioid agonists for NAS (Kaltenbach et al., 2012; Seligman et al., 2008). A pregnant woman's

opioid agonist dose should be increased as necessary to manage withdrawal and cravings. It should be expected that a pregnant woman will require increasing agonist doses across her pregnancy as her body volume and metabolism increase.

What affects NAS?

Maternal cigarette smoking (Jones et al., 2013) is associated with both increased risk of newborns needing opioid agonists for NAS (Kaltenbach et al., 2012) and birth defects like cleft lip and cleft palate (Cnattingius, 2004). Also, quitting smoking during treatment for opioid use disorder does not disrupt the opioid use disorder treatment (Dunn, Sigmon, Reimann, Heil, & Higgins, 2009). Thus, addressing tobacco use as part of medication-assisted treatment during pregnancy has significant health improvement potential.

Maternal use of selective serotonin reuptake inhibitors (SSRIs) can also increase the severity of NAS and length of treatment (Kaltenbach et al., 2012). Untreated maternal depression has its own detrimental effects on maternal and child health, so the risks and benefits of initiating or discontinuing SSRI use must be carefully considered.

Maternal benzodiazepine use also increases NAS severity and length of treatment (Seligman et al., 2008). Co-use of benzodiazepines and opioids greatly increases the risk of overdose and overdose death; thus, it is generally advisable to help co-users cease and abstain from benzodiazepine use. Benzodiazepine withdrawal can be dangerous, so gradual reductions in dose are usually necessary to avoid potentially fatal seizures. Inpatient withdrawal management is more successful than outpatient tapers.

Postpartum Considerations

Breastfeeding is generally appropriate and beneficial for the newborn when the mother is receiving opioid agonists as part of treatment. The American Academy of Pediatrics policy on breastfeeding states that a mother who uses illicit drugs (e.g., phencyclidine and cocaine) and cannabis should not breastfeed, nor should a mother with HIV or other specific rare health problems (Eidelman et al., 2012). Hepatitis C infection is not a contraindication for breastfeeding.

The postpartum period can be extremely stressful due to lost sleep and other life changes that come with having a newborn. Mothers with opioid use disorder are at increased risk for postpartum depression and should be monitored closely, using tools like the Edinburgh Postnatal Depression Scale (Holbrook & Kaltenbach, 2012). The stresses associated with the postpartum period may also trigger relapses, so careful continued monitoring and support are necessary.

Developmental Effects of Prenatal Opioid Exposure

There have been no consistent reports of developmental problems among children directly associated with prenatal opioid exposure. The longest and most comprehensive study of child development following opioid exposure to date found no substantive differences across 37 measures of physical and cognitive development between children exposed to methadone or buprenorphine during gestation, and development was on-par with the general population norms for all assessments (Kaltenbach et al., 2018).

Summary

Methadone or buprenorphine maintenance combined with comprehensive counseling and behavioral health care is the recommended standard care for pregnant women with opioid use. Replacement of illicitly-obtained opioids with these prescribed medications reduces risks of infections, such as Hepatitis B and C, HIV, and other infections that could be transmitted to the fetus or otherwise jeopardize the pregnancy.

Generally, opioid agonists used for medication-assisted treatment are safe for both maternal and infant health. It is also important to remember that Neonatal Abstinence Syndrome is a temporary and manageable condition. Furthermore, maternal cigarette smoking, untreated maternal depression, and benzodiazepine usage are important considerations to address within treatment, as these can be dangerous for both the mother and child.

4: Risks Associated with MMT
Emily Loscalzo, PsyD

Despite the many benefits of methadone maintenance, there are also risks associated with this treatment. It is important to learn how to talk to patients about these potential dangers, especially since there are so many myths associated with MMT. Coming into the therapeutic relationship armed with fact-based information can help with rapport-building and empowering the individual to become informed about the work you do with them.

General Side Effects

It is possible to experience side effects on methadone. For example, people who take methadone may experience unwanted effects such as sweating, constipation, drowsiness, decreased sexual desire or ability, or weight gain besides the therapeutic effects of treatment with this medication. Sometimes, there may be antidotes for some of these side effects or the dose can be adjusted to ensure continued therapeutic effects while reversing the side effects. These pharmacological antidotes may not be appropriate in all instances and other medications or antidotes may be available, so it is important for program participants to discuss all side effects with their prescribing physician to develop a plan to combat them. Here, we will go into greater detail about the most common side effects.

Sweating

Excessive sweating following initiation of methadone maintenance is thought to result from dysregulation of central thermoregulatory mechanisms (Catflisch et al., 2003) and/or mast cell degranulation (Gutstein & Akil, 2001). Many individuals on methadone maintenance are able to cope with this side effect; however, if it is very troublesome or interfering with daily functioning, biperiden, an anticholinergic (Catflisch et al., 2003), or desloratidine, an antihistamine (Al-Adwani & Basu, 2004) have been used as antidotes with some success.

Constipation

Due to the opioid effect of slowing peristalsis in the intestines, an increase in water absorption and a decrease in fluid and electrolyte secretion, opioid-induced constipation is frequently an issue. Recently, the standard of care is use of peripherally-acting μ-opioid receptor antagonists; that is, drugs that act by releasing some of the opioids from intestines and other peripheral organs, but not the brain to avoid increased craving and return to substance use. Naldemefdine (Stern & Brenner, 2018), methylnaltrexone (Chumpitz-Corredor & Lara-Solares, 2012), and naloxegol (Chey et al., 2014) are three such options used to offset this side effect. Other options exist, such as bisacodyl and sodium picosulfate (Muller-Lissner et al., 2017), senna (Feudtner et al., 2014), and other over-the-counter laxatives.

Drowsiness

Since methadone, like other opioids, depresses the central nervous system, not surprisingly, methadone may cause drowsiness. Rather than self-medicate with illicit substances, it may be effective for an individual to time their daily dose in such a way to decrease the likelihood of extreme drowsiness. This strategy may include taking the dose at a particular time of day or avoiding taking other medications that may cause drowsiness around the same time that methadone is taken. Excessive drowsiness also may be a signal that the dose is too high or too low or that the individual is using other sedating substances (i.e., benzodiazepines, other opioids) while on methadone. Therefore, it is imperative to check in with the prescribing physician if the drowsiness is particularly bothersome to the individual or if they are observed being extremely drowsy or "nodding off" while in session.

Decreased sexual desire or ability

This side effect is frequently a result of an increase in prolactin that decreases dopamine activity. Medications to decrease prolactin, such as bromocriptine, may work to counteract this side effect (Shinderman & Maxwell, 2000). The individual also may be experiencing relational issues or performance anxiety, particularly in early recovery. Couples or sex therapy may be a helpful supplement to their services in those instances.

Weight gain

MMT is associated with clinically significant weight gain. At times, this weight gain is welcome, as some individuals will enter treatment being significantly underweight. Methadone treatment with a proper diet can help them get their weight into the normal range. However, this may not always be the case, as many individuals will enter treatment at a healthy weight or beyond and find they are gaining additional weight since beginning methadone maintenance. Some studies suggest this phenomenon is particularly common among female patients (Fenn et al., 2014), while others state that males struggle more (Kolarzyk et al., 2005).

There is also some disagreement in the field on what the exact mechanism is behind the weight gain. Does methadone itself slow metabolism or cause increased cravings for sugar? Or is the increased food intake symptomatic of an addictive disorder, demonstrating that individuals who become abstinent from substance use shift the behavior to eating instead? A specific mechanism remains unknown; however, much of the literature so far supports that individuals who take methadone experience higher cravings and preference for sugary foods (Bogucka-Bonikowska et al., 2002; Nolan & Scagnelli, 2007; Zador, Wall, & Webster, 1996), which may be related to issues with glycemic control (Mysels & Sullivan, 2010). Genetics also seem to play a role, as certain changes in genetic material on the μ-opioid receptor are associated with binge-eating disorder and behaviors (Davis et al., 2009).

In terms of antidotes, the first line of defense should be conventional methods, such as diet and exercise. Individuals should work with their physicians on a healthy and sustainable weight loss plan (or better yet, a plan to prevent weight gain that is put into place when the individual begins treatment). Working with the physician is particularly important if the individual has other chronic health conditions. If the weight gain is already significant or if chronic health conditions prevent the individual from losing excess weight through conventional means, their physician may consider pharmacological antidotes to facilitate weight loss, such a topiramate, which has been shown to aid weight loss significantly as compared to placebo in individuals on MMT (Umbricht et al., 2015).

Risk of Overdose

Methadone may also present an increased risk of opioid overdose sometimes. Taking too much methadone could cause the individual to overdose on methadone, while too little methadone could leave the individual in withdrawal and therefore vulnerable to use other opioids. Helping the individual to work with their physician to find the proper dose is important.

The individual should also be warned that once they are on the right methadone dose, they can still overdose if they use other opioids. If an individual is prescribed an opioid after a medical procedure or in anesthesia, they must inform their treating physician they are taking methadone and inform the physician prescribing the methadone they will be receiving other opioids, so dosages can be adjusted, if necessary. Ideally, the individual should also allow both prescribing physicians to speak directly in order to most effectively coordinate their care and ensure the safest outcome.

Individuals may be more prone to overdose if they experience certain pre-existing conditions, such as liver or respiratory disease. If the liver is having more difficulty clearing out opioids due to disease, then individuals may experience prolonged exposure to opioids that may cause toxicity. The respiratory system may be adversely affected if it is already compromised, which could lead the individual to stop breathing.

Using benzodiazepines and other central nervous system depressants should also be avoided when taking methadone. These combinations can cause a synergistic effect; that is, an effect greater than the sum of each medication's individual effect. In the United

States, fatalities from such combinations are on the rise, with benzodiazepine deaths involving opioids increasing six-fold more than those not involving opioids (NIDA, 2018a).

Withdrawal

Precipitous withdrawal from methadone can be harmful, particularly when individuals relapse on opioids or have preexisting medical conditions.

Relapse on opioids during withdrawal
When an individual is tapering off methadone, they may be more likely to relapse on opioids in order to self-medicate withdrawal symptoms. Particularly with illicit Schedule I substances such as heroin, this relapse can be dangerous. As mentioned in Chapter 1, heroin may be laced with any number of other substances, from rat poison to fentanyl to carfentanil. Those extraneous substances alone can be fatal. With the individual's lowered tolerance due to the decreased methadone dose, illicit opioids are even more dangerous. Individuals may also overestimate their tolerance and accidentally overdose.

Preexisting medical conditions
Due to the risks associated with abrupt cessation of MMT, individuals should be decreased on their methadone dose gradually (10mg per week until 40mg is reached; 5mg per week thereafter). Individuals may taper off methadone more rapidly, but it is not recommended (WHO, 2009). Involuntary detoxification may be indicated if the individual's behavior threatens the health and/or safety of others, but

this measure should only be taken as a last resort (WHO, 2009). It is not recommended that pregnant women taper off methadone due to possible danger to the developing baby. If a woman chooses to taper off methadone during her pregnancy, she should not start until after the first trimester and the taper should be only 2.5 to 5mg per week (WHO, 2009). Death is otherwise possible in withdrawal from opioids, including methadone, if persistent vomiting and diarrhea occur and are left untreated, as these symptoms may cause dehydration, hypernatremia, and heart failure (Darke, Larney, & Farrell, 2017). Individuals with pre-existing heart conditions and seizure disorders should avoid rapid detoxification from methadone due to these potentially fatal complications.

Driving

In general, it is considered safe to drive while on methadone maintenance, regardless of dosage, provided that the dosage is not too high for the individual taking it; performance decreases considerably when alcohol and/or benzodiazepines are taken with methadone (Chesher et al., 1989). When dose adjustments occur, it is safest for the individual on methadone maintenance to avoid driving until they understand how the dose adjustment has affected them.

Methadone Diversion

Concern about methadone doses being diverted is significant. To help avoid dispensed doses from being diverted by either patients or staff, methadone maintenance programs are required to establish a diversion control plan for accreditation. There are a number of aspects involved in a diversion control plan. Many rules and regulations of opioid treatment programs, including elements of a diversion control plan are developed with patient safety at the forefront.

It may help both the counselor and the individual in treatment to view the rules and regulations from the perspective of safety. These policies were put in place to protect the safety of the individuals we are serving as treatment providers. It is also important to provide individuals seeking treatment with this information before they join the program, so they can be aware of rules and regulations of the program and consent to them before they begin.

Below are some of the safeguards that are put into place at most programs to ensure that the methadone dispensed to each individual is used by that individual only, and to prevent the methadone from being diverted to individuals who are not the intended patient. This is not meant to be an exhaustive list of such safeguards; consult with your program director and have a strong understanding of your agency's policies.

- All urine drug screens given by patients are observed by staff members, usually nursing staff, through closed-circuit cameras (or direct observation, if necessary). **Urine samples** are then checked by nurses for color and temperature. If it is discovered that a program participant has submitted another individual's urine or another substance other than urine during a drug screen (also known as adulteration), many programs will have the participant leave the program (usually after repeated adulteration despite being informed of rules against this behavior). This rule results from the concern that the urine drug screens are being adulterated to mask diversion.

- **Oral drug screens** may be used instead of urine drug screening occasionally, depending on state regulations. This type of drug screen may be more challenging to adulterate and therefore could detect diversion or minimize the risk of diversion by acting as a deterrent.
- Drug screens always test for methadone and its metabolite, 2-ethylidene-1,5-dimethyl-3,3-diphenylpyrrolidine **(EDDP)**. The test for methadone is performed to ensure that the program participant is, indeed, positive for methadone; further, the EDDP metabolite test to ensure that the individual is actually ingesting the substance. Specifically, EDDP is the molecule made after the individual ingests methadone and their body breaks down the drug, and it is what is excreted in the urine. Therefore, individuals must be positive for both methadone and EDDP to determine that they are ingesting their methadone dose each day. Drug testing for other illicit substances and their metabolites is also essential for methadone diversion control, client safety, and informing treatment direction.
- Using a state's **Prescription Drug Monitoring Program (PDMP)**, an internet database that physicians search when prescribing controlled substances (i.e., benzodiazepines, opioids, etc.) to determine what other controlled substances a patient is prescribed, which physician(s) are prescribing it, and the date and quantity of the substance they are picking up. This database is a tool to ensure safety and to encourage coordination of care between physicians.
- For program participants without take-home privileges, their methadone must be taken at the medicating window every

day (in most states), in full view of the medicating staff. Individuals with take-home privileges must also follow this procedure on the days of the week they are medicated at the clinic and when called for a take-home bottle callback. **Speaking after the dose is swallowed ensures that individuals are ingesting their full dose**, rather than holding it in their mouths so they may spit it out or otherwise transfer it to another individual.

- Patients who have earned take-home privileges are required to return the same bottle, empty, to the medicating nurse upon returning to the clinic for medication every time they receive take-home bottle(s).
    o **Take-home bottle callbacks** are another method of diversion control. In most states, callbacks are required for individuals receiving 3 or more consecutive take-home bottles. The general procedure involves nursing staff members calling the individual and asking them to return to the clinic during business hours the same day. At this time, the nursing staff ensures that the individual has the expected number of full and empty take-home bottles and expects the full bottles to ensure that they were not tampered with. They will usually send one or more of the full bottles to the lab to be tested for **methadone integrity**: is the substance in the bottle methadone, and does it contain the expected number of milligrams of methadone? This procedure ensures that the medication is being taken as prescribed. If any aspect of the take-home callback process goes awry (including being unable to reach the

individual by phone), then take-home privileges are suspended for a period of time, and sometimes indefinitely, depending on the severity of the concerns of the physician.
- During periods when many patients will be given take-home bottles, such as a **weather emergency**, the local police are usually notified so that they may provide more frequent patrols of the area around the clinic to ensure that methadone is not being diverted.

Methadone diversion is taken seriously, as methadone is a very potent substance that could lead to abuse, overdose, or death, particularly in individuals who have not developed a tolerance for opioids. Program participants and staff members alike who are caught trying to divert methadone from a program are handled using disciplinary policies, which usually include discharge or termination from the program.

Summary

Methadone is a useful medication that is highly effective in treating opioid use disorder. However, the various risks associated with its use must be considered when admitting and maintaining an individual in a program. Counselors can empower their clients by educating them about side effects, risks associated with overdose and withdrawal, and program policies, particularly about diversion control. The counselor can also act as the liaison between the client and the program physicians to ensure that they are getting the medical and psychiatric help they need, managing side effects, and avoiding life-threatening risks while in methadone maintenance treatment.

5: Harm Reduction

*"Although the world is full of suffering,
it is full also of the overcoming of it."*
– Helen Keller

Harm reduction is a controversial and humanitarian attitude towards reducing the physical injury associated with high-risk behaviors (Marlatt, Larimer, & Witkiewitz, 2011). This is counter to prevailing models of abstinence-based or drug-free treatment. Harm reduction has a strong commitment to public health and human rights (Harm Reduction International, 2017).

It is not necessarily a specific set of rules or regulations, but rather a perspective seeking to improve the overall quality of life for individuals, and the communities they live in (Harm Reduction Coalition, as cited by Marlatt, Larimer, & Witkiewitz, 2011). This view of preserving life and reducing injury is central to the methadone maintenance model.

MMT and Harm Reduction

In theory, methadone treatment is utilized to replace the harmful and illicit opioid(s) that a client is using. According to the National Center for Health Statistics, there were 64,070 reported drug overdose deaths during a 12-month period in 2016. This is a 21% increase compared to totals compiled from 2015 (National Center for Health Statistics, 2017).

With the overall "cut" or concoction (as discussed in Chapters 1 and 4) of heroin becoming increasingly adulterated, not surprisingly, more people are dying from accidental overdoses every year.

Though abstinence may be a goal for clients at some later point in their future recovery, it is imperative we respect the client's autonomy and "meet them where they are at." This also honors the prospect that a participant may never want to elicit complete abstinence from all substances.

As previously cited, research suggests that methadone maintenance provides decreased illicit opioid use and better treatment retention compared to non-opioid replacement programs (Ball & Ross, 2012; Connock et al., 2007; Marsch, 1998; Mattick, Breen, Kimber, & Davoli, 2009). From the perspective of reducing physical injury to a client, MMT can also reduce rates of mortality, additional contact with the criminal justice system, and rates of hepatitis C infection (Dolan et al., 2005).

Finally, it is important to note that methadone is a prescribed medication strictly regulated at a state and federal level for opioid addiction. At least in the United States, methadone can only be prescribed as a part of maintenance within a treatment setting.

Overdose Education and Response

Opioid-related overdose can often be witnessed through losing consciousness, unresponsiveness to stimulus, inability to communicate, slow/shallow/erratic breathing (or lack thereof), purple/gray skin tones, choking noises, vomiting, blue/purple fingernails and lips, and slow pulse (Harm Reduction Coalition, 2018b).

It is encouraged that providers help educate participants on what to look for in a potential opioid-related overdose: the importance of calling for help by dialing emergency medical services, how to place the victim in a recovery position (laying their body and face on their side, with their body supported by a bent knee), and how to get connected to a local training on administering naloxone and basic life support.

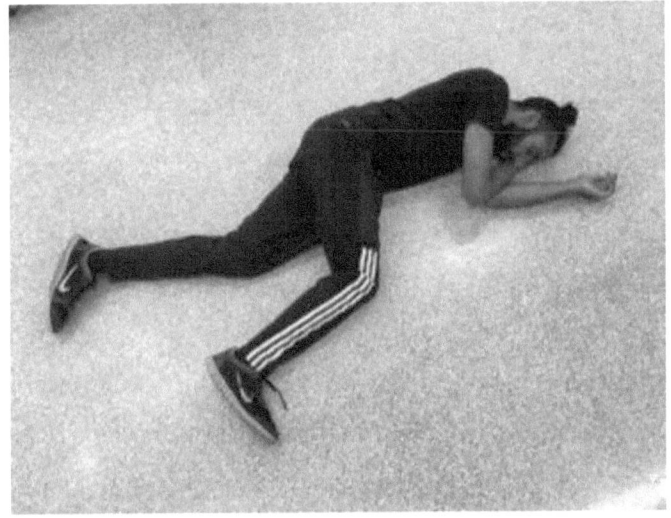

Figure 4. The recovery position.

Naloxone (the popular nasal spray is called Narcan®) is an opioid antagonist considered an "antidote" that reverses the effects of an accidental overdose and allows emergency responders to intervene and potentially save a life. It can generally work within 2-3 minutes, and additional dosages can be administered until emergency medical assistance arrives; one dosage may not be enough. It stays in the body for about 2 hours (Narcan®, 2017).

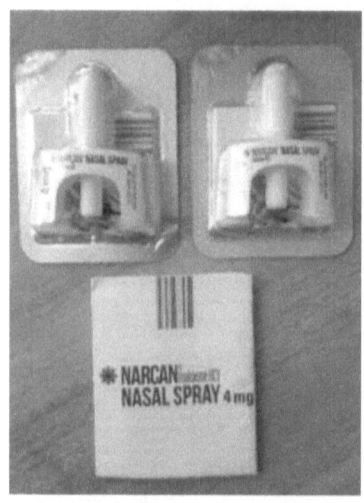

Figure 5. Two 4 mg Narcan® nasal sprays.

Narcan® is offered over the counter in 46 states from a standing order through the Physician's General (Caruso, 2017). It can be covered by commercial insurance or state-funded insurance. There is a large misconception that creating access to this medication in urban areas leads to more illicit substance use. Research has demonstrated that the prescription of naloxone does not encourage people to use opioids more (Seal et al., 2003).

Along with carrying naloxone as a tool for overdose response, clients may also opt to not use substances alone to help provide additional support if a peer is showing the signs of potential overdose.

Provision of Medical and Psychiatric Services

At a federal level in the United States, opioid treatment programs are required to "provide adequate medical, counseling, vocational, educational, and other assessment and treatment services" (SAMHSA, 2015). Although a client may initially come seeking relief from withdrawal symptoms from opioids through methadone stabilization, the treatment setting can also lend itself to providing additional services to help improve client quality of life.

Services may also include additional psychiatric assessment and medication management, referrals for adjunctive therapies, and referrals for primary care. Given the prevalence of hepatitis C and HIV among those that are injection drug users (Hagan, Thiede, & Des Jarlais, 2005), medical attention and possible pharmacological intervention for infectious diseases and other health complications can improve overall clinical outcomes for our clients.

Referrals to Appropriate Levels of Care

A treatment facility may offer a continuum of services ranging from ambulatory detoxification up to medically managed residential treatment services. Mental health providers can serve as facilitators within requests for additional funding for alternative levels of care, based on placement criteria (i.e., ASAM, or assessment tools unique to the state where you are practicing, like the Pennsylvania Client Placement Criteria (PCPC).

Summary

When we adopt an attitude and perspective grounded in harm reduction, we are focused on preserving life and limiting the amount of physical injury that an individual is enacting on themselves and others.

Methadone maintenance is a form of medication-assisted treatment dedicated to dialing back the harm inherent within the potential chronic nature of relapse in addiction. It is the hope that this treatment allows an individual to regain a sense of stability in their lives while rebuilding their health, relationships, and livelihood.

With drug overdose as now the leading cause of death for Americans under the age of 50, it is crucial to act. By providing the needed education and tools for both treatment providers and the public, we are anticipating the prospect of fatality in drug use and trying to prevent it.

6: Trauma and Chemical Dependency

*"There is no greater agony than bearing
an untold story inside of you."*
– Maya Angelou

When we experience pain, there is a natural tendency to want to find a way to relieve it. Literature suggests that clients who experience trauma-related distress often use alcohol and drugs in a problematic way (Brady, Back, & Coffey 2004; Ouimette & Brown, 2003). If the identifiable stressor and the pain associated with it are not addressed within treatment, it could be argued that continued substance use will remain as the client's most familiar coping skill.

The Adverse Childhood Experiences Study (ACE Study) is an investigation conducted by Kaiser Permanente and the U.S. Centers for Disease Control and Prevention. Its findings demonstrated that individuals with five or more ACEs reported are seven to ten times more likely to report illicit drug use. If six or more ACEs are reported, a person is a staggering 46 times more likely to use intravenous drugs than those who report no ACEs (Felitti et al., 1998).

A potential connection between experienced trauma-related distress and coping through the use of substances can bring insight and awareness into a client's understanding of their condition. It is important to employ culturally sensitive screening and assessment tools to help best identify what challenge areas are causing the most distress for a client. Several popular screening instruments include the Primary Care PTSD Screen for DSM-5 (PC-PTSD-5), SPAN, SPRINT, and Trauma Screening Questionnaire (TSQ) (U.S. Department of Veterans Affairs, 2017a). Additionally, it is worthy to note that the recent validation of the International Trauma Questionnaire (ITQ) brings promise to diagnosing PTSD and complex PTSD (Hyland et al., 2017). A list of all measures can be found at https://www.ptsd.va.gov/professional/assessment/all_measures.asp.

Following a thorough screening and assessment for trauma-related distress, a clinician can help collaboratively formulate a treatment plan utilizing the best evidence-based practices that can provide the most relief to a participant.

We will initially explore the stages of trauma recovery as detailed by Herman (1992). Following this, we will examine a brief overview and ways to deepen a study of three of the most well-supported forms of treating PTSD. The intention is to maximize the ways to help clients on your caseload who may be experiencing challenges relating to trauma.

Evidence-Based Treatments for PTSD

The U.S. National Center for Posttraumatic Stress Disorder (PTSD) promotes three types of trauma-focused therapies that have had a number of clinical outcome trials conducted to evaluate their effectiveness in treating PTSD. These are Prolonged Exposure (PE), Cognitive Processing Therapy (CPT), and Eye-Movement Desensitization and Reprocessing (EMDR) (U.S. Department of Veterans Affairs, 2017b). A brief overview of each treatment plus ways to deepen the study of them are offered.

It important to mention that this chapter is not meant to be a complete list of all approaches to treating traumatic distress, but rather a way to stimulate personal and professional research into possible instruments to put into your toolbox. There are many different types of trauma-informed approaches, and as Herman (1992) states, "There is no single, efficacious "magic bullet" for the traumatic syndromes." What may bring relief for one client may not work for another.

SAMHSA defines a trauma-informed approach as one that:

- "*Realizes* the widespread impact of trauma and understands potential paths for recovery."
- "*Recognizes* the signs and symptoms of trauma in clients, families, staff, and others involved with the system."
- "*Responds* by fully integrating knowledge about trauma into policies, procedures, and practices."
- "Seeks to actively resist *re-traumatization*."

It is best practice to respect the survivor and keep them informed, connected, and hopeful about their recovery. Working with survivors to collaborate with their families and other social supports is also important (SAMHSA, 2018).

Herman's Stages of Trauma Recovery

The goal of Judith Herman's influential three-stage approach to trauma recovery is to establish safety and stability, explore and mourn the losses associated with the trauma, and then cultivate the survivor's internal and external resources to aid them in achieving a new post-traumatic life (Herman, 1992).

The following is a basic overview of some key components within each stage:

Stage 1: Establish safety

- There is the development of a strong therapeutic alliance.
- A thorough and informed diagnostic evaluation is completed.
- Survivor power and control is restored.
- There is an establishment of bodily and environmental safety.
- Awareness of symptom recognition and comprehension of the effect of trauma is built.
- Meaning making surrounding body sensations, intrusive emotions and distorted cognitive schemas is created.
- Emotional stability through coping skill development to manage triggered symptoms is developed.
- Medication management is utilized, if needed and agreeable to the survivor.

Stage 2: Remembrance and mourning

- Once there is safety established, the survivor tells and re-tells the story of the trauma completely with depth and detail to the mental health professional.
- There is a reconstruction of the trauma, including the survivor's life before the trauma and the circumstances that led to the event, traumatic imagery, bodily sensations and the responses of the survivor plus their support system to the trauma.
- Safety and stabilization are re-established if the client becomes overwhelmed and intrusions become pervasive.

- A systematic review of the meaning of the event is co-constructed.
- Loss from the trauma is mourned, allowing for a space where the client can grieve.

Stage 3: Reconnection and integration

- Power in real-life situations is reclaimed as well as active engagement with their world.
- There is a re-creation of the ideal self.
- Healthy attachments are established.
- There is work toward personal and professional goals congruent with post-traumatic growth.
- Survivors are reminded that recovery is an on-going process.

Where can I learn more about the Phases of Trauma Recovery?

1. **Self-study:** please see *Trauma and Recovery: The Aftermath of Violence-From Domestic Abuse to Political Terror* by Judith Herman. ISBN-13: 978-0465061716
2. **Peer learning group and case consultation.**

Prolonged Exposure Therapy (PE)

PE is like Herman's work, as it is rooted in a client telling, retelling and listening to the self-recounting of the trauma with an underlying goal of confronting the trauma. It was developed by Edna B. Foa, PhD, the acting director of the Center for the Treatment and Study of Anxiety at the University of Pennsylvania.

PE has been empirically supported with helping to reduce the symptoms of PTSD, depression, anger, and anxiety in trauma survivors; it has been an effective form of treatment with those suffering from substance dependency and PTSD when combined with concurrent chemical dependency treatment (CTSA, 2018a).

PE is a structured cognitive behavioral therapy that lasts eight to fifteen sessions, either weekly or twice-weekly. Each session is 90 minutes. The CTSA states that sessions include elements of "discussing frightening thoughts, breathing retraining, confronting safe situations, and/or by revisiting and recounting painful memories in order to process them and reduce their emotional impact" (CTSA, 2018b).

Where can I learn more about PE?

1. **Self-study**: please see *Prolonged Exposure Therapy for PTSD: Emotional Processing of Traumatic Experiences (Treatments That Work)* by Edna B. Foa, Elizabeth A. Hembree, and Barbara Olaslov Rothbaum ISBN-13: 978-0195308501 as well as *Reclaiming Your Life from a Traumatic Experience: A Prolonged Exposure Treatment Program (Treatments That Work) by Barbara Olaslov Rothbaum,* Edna B. Foa, and Elizabeth A. Hembree. ISBN-13: 978-0195308488
2. **Formal training:** attend a 4-day intensive workshop conducted by the Center for the Treatment and Study of Anxiety.
3. **Consultation:** collaborate with certified PE consultants accredited by the Center for the Treatment and Study of Anxiety.

Cognitive Processing Therapy (CPT)

CPT is a cognitive behavioral therapy (CBT) treatment that primarily focuses on the connections between thoughts, feelings, body sensations, and behaviors associated with PTSD and related conditions.

A course of treatment lasts for twelve 50-minute therapy sessions, where the content is described by its authors as "getting information on common reactions to trauma, identifying and challenging unhelpful thoughts with structured therapy sessions, and completing regular out-of-session practice assignments to apply what has been discussed in therapy sessions."

More specifically, topics within sessions cover "the meaning of the traumatic event(s), identification of thoughts and feelings, trust issues, safety issues, issues of power and control, esteem issues, and intimacy issues" (Cognitive Processing Therapy for PTSD, n.d.).

Where can I learn more about CPT?

1. **Self-study:** please see *Cognitive Processing Therapy for PTSD: A Comprehensive Manual by* Patricia A. Resick, Candice M. Monson, and Kathleen M. Chard. ISBN-13: 978-1462528646
2. **Formal training:** attend workshops endorsed by the treatment authors, which can be located on the official CPT website. Additionally, https://cpt.musc.edu/index offers a 9-hour web-based training. It was developed by the National Crime Victims Research and Treatment Center at the Medical University of South Carolina in collaboration with the National Center for PTSD.

3. **Consultation:** Individual and group consultation via telephone are available to licensed mental health providers that have completed CPTweb and a live CPT training (2-3 days) conducted by a treatment developer or an approved CPT Trainer.

Eye Movement Desensitization and Reprocessing Therapy (EMDR)

EMDR is an integrative psychotherapy developed by Francine Shapiro, PhD to treat PTSD in 1987 (Shapiro, 2001). Treatment consists of six to twelve weekly or twice-weekly sessions. A length of treatment may differ based on the number of traumas and when the PTSD was onset (EMDR Institute, Inc., 2018).

Sessions are focused on having the patient focus directly on the traumatic memory while being bilaterally stimulated, most commonly through eye movements; this stimulation can also be achieved using tones or taps with a device specifically engineered for the same purpose.

The use of bilateral stimulation is to induce a neurobiological state similar to rapid eye movement (REM) sleep, which may reintegrate how traumatic memories are stored (Stickgold, 2002). During EMDR the focus is on transforming the emotional experiences that a trauma survivor has experienced, as evidenced by a client's thoughts, feelings, and behaviors following reprocessing.

A detailed overview of the eight phases of treatment can be found on the EMDR Institute, Inc. website at http://www.emdr.com/what-is-emdr/.

Where can I learn more about EMDR?

1. **Self-study:** please see *Eye Movement Desensitization and Reprocessing (EMDR) Therapy, Third Edition: Basic Principles, Protocols, and Procedures* by Francine Shapiro. ISBN-13: 978-1462532766
2. **Formal training:** attend The EMDR Therapy Basic Training (Weekend 1 and 2) through the EMDR Institute, Inc.
3. **Consultation:** collaborate with EMDR Institute approved consultants.

Summary

These are a few well-respected and evidence-based practices for problems resulting from trauma. With every individual that walks through our doors, it is integral to consider the possible role that trauma has had within the development of chemical dependency, given the substantial evidence that suggests there is a connection.

With all these therapies used to address PTSD and other types of distress from trauma, clinicians must receive appropriate training before using these techniques and remember to work within their professional abilities.

It is also not to say these are the only tried-and-true ways to alleviate distress from trauma. Every client we work with has been through distinct experiences that have made them uniquely themselves. It is necessary that we constantly evaluate and re-evaluate why a modality may or may not work for our participants.

7: Motivational Interviewing

Change is difficult for all humans. For those dealing with chemical dependency, it is especially challenging to readily embrace it. There has never been a client I have worked with who openly said that they enjoyed being dependent on substances and wanted to stay in the position they were in. Our participants know that continuing to expose themselves to drugs has meaningful consequences.

Change is hard, and I commend every client that has walked through our doors on wanting to try. It takes a great deal of courage and vulnerability to admit that something is not right and attempt to make things better. Given that substance addiction is a chronic medical condition (McLellan, Lewis, O'brien, & Kleber, 2000) that is progressive in nature, every participant's recovery process looks different because they are at varying stages of change.

The Stages of Change

Gauging where a client is at in their recovery is a good way to get an initial benchmark and collaboratively determine how to get to where they want to be. Below is an illustration of the Transtheoretical Model of Change (Prochaska & DiClemente, 1982), which can be a useful tool for making this assessment.

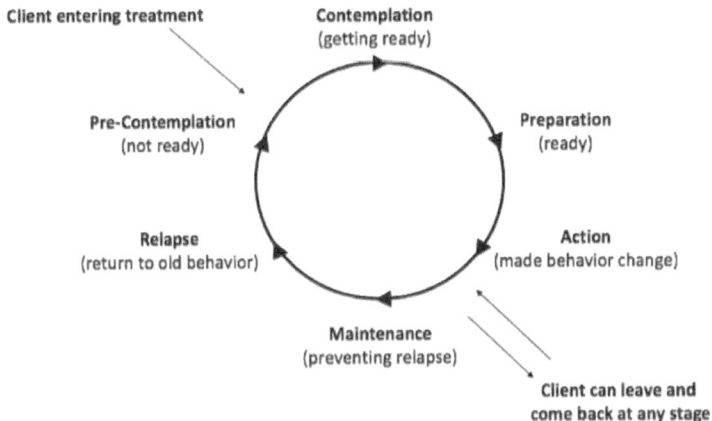

Figure 6. An illustration of the Transtheoretical Model of Change (1982).

Within this model, a client may enter treatment at varying degrees of motivation or leave and return at distinct points. In examining what factors are leaving clients ambivalent to change, there is a way of speaking to them called Motivational Interviewing (MI) that helps to clarify and guide towards an intended behavior.

What is Motivational Interviewing (MI)?

It is an evidenced-based clinical method that is effective in resolving ambivalence towards client change. As a service provider, it can be a powerful style of communication (Miller & Rollnick, 2009) that aids in improving program engagement by increasing participant motivation and commitment to transformative aspects of recovery.

It is important to know that there is an overarching "spirit," or manner in which this communicational style is used, that incorporates partnership, acceptance, compassion, and evocation. These client-centered principles help guide the steps needed for change. In

Motivational Interviewing: Helping People Change (3rd ed.), Miller and Rollnick (2012) outline these four processes:

1. **Engaging:** establishing a helpful connection and working relationship.
2. **Focusing:** clarifying the direction of what changes the client hopes for.
3. **Evoking:** eliciting the client's own motivations for change.
4. **Planning:** developing a commitment to change and formulating a specific plan of action.

Assessing Readiness to Change

When assessing clients for how ready they are to change, it is crucial to gather more information about the level of importance for them, as well as how confident they think that they are in making this change.

Scaling questions, such as "how important is it to you to ___?" from 0-10 can help provide this information about *importance*. Additionally, "how confident are you that you could ___, if you decided to?" offers more surrounding the participant's *confidence* to change this behavior.

```
How important is this change to you right now?
0   1   2   3   4   5   6   7   8   9   10
Not             Somewhat         Very
```

```
How confident are you about making this change?
0   1   2   3   4   5   6   7   8   9   10
Not             Somewhat         Very
```

Figure 7. Readiness Rulers.

A *Readiness Ruler* is a tool that is easy to create and can help stream-line the conversation about planning for and beginning change in a tangible way. It consists of one strip of paper that asks the client from 0-10, "how important is this change for you right now?" and another strip of paper that asks from 0-10, "how confident are you about making this change?" (Center for Evidence-Based Practices, 2010).

Exploring Client Change with O.A.R.S.

Categorically, MI is client-centered. It operates within an empathetic and non-judgmental space. In establishing this safe environment, four client-centered strategies illustrated by the acronym "O.A.R.S." are used early and often. Rollnick (2002) describes this abbreviation as standing for:

- **O**pen-ended questions: these cannot be answered with a "yes" or "no" response, "what has worked in the past when you have felt triggered?"
- **A**ffirmations: identifying a personal strength evidenced by what the client has shown, "John, it took a great deal of courage to come in today."
- **R**eflective listening: this is reflecting back a client's thoughts, feelings, and behaviors, "you're feeling sad because you've been thinking about the break-up" or "I noticed that you clenched your fists when you spoke about your brother, what are you feeling right now?"
- **S**ummaries: Giving a condensed version of what the client has shared with you. More broadly, this is asking the question of

whether you heard the client correctly, "It sounds like you've been troubled by what your partner expressed to you last night. Although both of you are committed to making things work in the relationship, it couldn't help but bring a sense of uncertainty that has felt frightening."

These communicational techniques help build rapport and safety, facilitate the development of insight, and allow a participant to view their situation in an alternative light.

"Change Talk" Versus "Sustain Talk"

MI is goal-oriented. A clinician partners with a client to help reconcile their own ambivalence towards objectives in treatment by eliciting the language of change. There is an emphasis on this particular type of communication, while curiously exploring what barriers may be hindering a client from reaching their treatment goals through O.A.R.S.

This language of change is referred to as "change talk" (e.g., "I want to cut down on my using"), which is contrasted with "sustain talk" ("but, I couldn't even if I tried"). Eliciting "change talk" through using O.A.R.S. can be like bowling a game with bumpers. Bumpers provide a physical barrier and guide by preventing the bowling ball from going into the gutter. Like these bumpers, we can help a client guide their own dialogue while clarifying desires for change through calculated conversation.

Research shows that such commitment language can predict behavioral change (Amrhein, Miller, Yahne, Palmer, & Fulcher, 2003; Amrhein, 2004). The more a participant utilizes this type of language to describe what they hope to accomplish, the more devotion there is to realize their treatment goals.

In summation, the collaborative plan for a mental health provider in Motivational Interviewing consists of assessing *importance* and *confidence* to change, recognizing "change talk," getting clients to interface more with it, and strategically guiding them to respond in a way that helps bring about behavioral change.

Where can I learn more about MI?

A. **Self-study:** please see *Motivational Interviewing* (3rd ed.) by William R. Miller and Stephen Rollnick. ISBN-13: 978-1609182274

B. **Motivational Interviewing peer learning group:** audio-record or videotape sessions and code with peer feedback. This can help create a learning plan for the clinician.

C. **Formal training:** attend trainings conducted by MINT (Motivational Interviewing Network of Trainers), and in-house facility trainings, if offered.

Summary

Motivational Interviewing can be a crucial style of communication with clients. With a natural person-centered approach, it "rolls with the ambivalence" that a client may have. Often, when we try to tell someone what they *should* or *should not* be doing, it can generate a wide array of negative emotions and undo the groundwork that was established in a safe and trusting therapeutic relationship.

If using MI, we are respecting the autonomy of a client, while naturally presenting their own reasons for possibly discontinuing a behavior causing them harm.

8: Involving Loved Ones in Treatment

There is a saying that "you can choose your friends, but you can't choose your family." Families are complicated and often, origin stories have the potential to help a participant make sense of another layer within their addiction. When conducting family sessions within MMT, counselors can serve several roles.

These may consist of providing psychoeducation surrounding the methadone maintenance process, identifying ways to emotionally support the client in a skillful manner, ushering in more sober social support, and helping to communicate the varying effects that addiction can have on the family system. It is important to note that the role of a substance use counselor differs from a family therapist, and it is imperative to refer out if providing family therapy is not in your professional scope of practice (CSAT, 2004a).

Family of Origin Considerations for Treating Chemical Dependency

Research suggests there are numerous genes that affect the risk for substance dependence (Dick & Agrawal, 2008; Renthal & Nestler, 2008). This biological predisposition could play a role within intergenerational addiction. In addition, the prospect for risk within developing this condition can also be partially mediated by parental factors like poor inhibitory control and poor discipline (Pears, Capaldi, & Owen, 2007). Early caregivers can play a significant factor in developing unhealthy coping strategies for clients.

Furthermore, the home could be a source of information that provides insight surrounding high-risk situations for potential resumed use. Sometimes a client may be actively engaging in substance use with their family or perceived intimate supports, plus in frequent contact with stress and conflict with who's at home. Or, perhaps their family members are providing a means of enabling the substance dependency to continue.

These morsels of information can help the client and treatment provider facilitate healthy lifestyle changes within the family system, even simply from fostering insight. Such modifications could aid in filling in gaps where a family has unmet needs or help fuel an interest in referrals to more appropriate levels of care, such as a residential program or halfway house.

The Role of Family Sessions in Treatment

A family session could serve as an opportunity to help provide education and stigma management surrounding the theory and practice of MMT, as well as the overarching disease model of addiction.

A client's support network may need to hear about the Phases of Treatment Model (Moolchan and Hoffman, 1994) aforementioned in Chapters 1 and 2, or even psychoeducation surrounding the disease model of addiction. Therefore, it is paramount to create a safe environment in which the client and family can attend to accurate information surrounding addiction, the role that methadone plays within MMT, and how they can best support their loved one.

Often, as a function of the disease of addiction, trust can be violated when a client acts to have their needs met. Clients may not be able to access the language or knowledge to help their loved ones understand what they need from them to support their recovery efforts, and how difficult it may be in the early stages of treatment to express these needs in healthy ways.

With individualized relapse prevention work, it might also be helpful to facilitate the conversation between the participant and their family members in providing the most appropriate support possible for treatment retention and success.

Triangulation and Why It Matters

The concept of *triangulation* in family therapy is most often connected with work by Murray Bowen (The Bowen Center, 2018). It is considered the smallest and most stable relationship system because it involves three people and can often build bigger interlocking emotional systems. Its stability is due to its nature in spreading tension across three people, rather than just two. During periods of calm in these relationships, two people will be comfortably close "insiders" and the third is an uncomfortable "outsider."

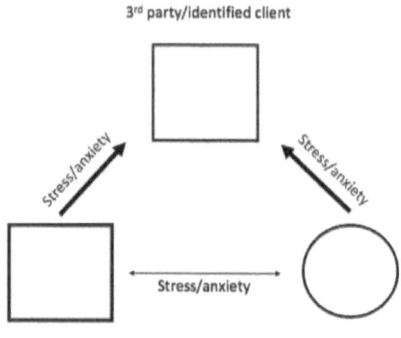

Dyad stress/anxiety is directed to 3rd party

Figure 8. A graphic example of triangulation with a mother, father, and a son.

When tension becomes too strong between two people, energy can be diverted to the third person or institution, which may be considered a go-between, scapegoat, object of concern, or ally (CSAT, 2004a). For example, between two parents, a child who is often the identified client can be pushed into an outsider position as a function of their condition or they may side with a parent they are closer with, forcing the other parent to be vilified.

Truth be told, mental health professionals can unknowingly be ushered into these dynamics if they do not utilize family sessions with the treatment regimen. For instance, a client may be torn between the expectations of their family and their treatment program, creating uninspired treatment engagement. Involving family members in treatment is essential to help alleviate this tension and ensure that all individuals involved in the client's treatment are on the same page.

Supporting the Family Through the Immediate Community

Self-help groups like *Al-Anon*, which focus on offering fellowship to those that have been affected by a loved one's addiction have been around since the 1950s (Al-Anon, 2016). While it can be important to include support groups within a participant's on-going treatment, it can also be equally valuable for family members to have their own support as well.

There is a ripple-effect with substance use. Depending on the client's social support network and their familiarity with addiction, it could generate an increased amount of stress and frustration that partially stems from what is not known about their loved one's condition.

Along with counseling, support groups for those affected by a loved one's addiction can be helpful for giving a sense of hope and connection. As with any support group, these spaces are a reminder that no one must go through their trials alone. See the "Useful Websites and Useful Books" sections for more tools to connect family and friends of those in recovery with.

Summary

Family systems are complicated, in as much as the addiction we are trying to treat. Including family members into substance use treatment can be a doorway into better understanding the challenges that both the client and their loved ones face when confronted with addiction.

In this sort of capacity, a methadone counselor can provide education into what addiction *is* and what *it is not*, the science surrounding MMT, help facilitate communication between the client and their loved ones, and link family members to the best sources of support. Within this role, it is integral to know your scope of practice, and to know your professional limitations within practicing family therapy.

9: Support

"It takes a village to raise a child."

– African Proverb

The quote above is an ancient African proverb that embodies the spirit of requiring many partnerships for a person to grow up in a safe environment. Depending on the way that MMT is regulated in your area, you may see a client for session once a week, or even less frequently than that. This is a minuscule fraction of the over 168 hours there are in a week, leaving room for change from outside the treatment environment.

Support from peers and professionals comes in many forms, whether within the treatment facility, from outside support groups, community-based agencies offering intensive case management services, or in web-based settings. No matter the source, it can help instill hope, build fellowship, and allow clients to feel understood as having a condition that does not define who they are.

An Overview of Peer Support

Although there are many roads to recovery, peer support can help provide clients a unique sense of belonging, connection, and purpose they may not directly receive through their treatment provider. Those that have lived the experience can give distinctive perspectives and an accurate understanding of what a client may be going through.

Potential options for clients looking to receive additional support from their peers may consist of choices from both inside the treatment facility and outside in the larger community. Regardless of where it is found, experts can agree that support is a necessity in the recovery process. Literature suggests that higher amounts of this recovery capital, such as social support and 12-step facilitation, can be predictors of positive outcomes across different stages of recovery (Laudet & White, 2008).

Support from Inside the Treatment Setting

In-house self-help meetings
A facility may host in-house self-help groups to develop community and provide an environment that individuals can bond and relate through a common thread of addiction. These may be closed to the larger community but facilitated by an individual in recovery.

Frequently enough, these meetings are often guided by those that have participated in a treatment program. These valuable perspectives and insights are something that a direct treatment provider cannot bring to the table like a peer can.

Professional peer support
Depending on county and state staffing requirements for drug and alcohol treatment, a treatment team may also include a nationally certified peer recovery support specialist (NCPRSS). Regionally, this professional may also be referred to as a certified peer specialist (CPS) or certified recovery specialist (CRS).

These are trained professionals that are integral for providing their lived experience to clients; they have self-identified as having a mental health challenge or may be in recovery themselves, respectively. This marriage between formal education and training plus lived experience can supply a unique skill set to any treatment team. Preliminary research suggests that peer-supported community programs can have a positive effect on community affiliation and supportive behaviors within giving and receiving help for substance use challenges (Boisvert, Martin, Grosek, & Clarie, 2008).

Certified peers can help a participant navigate a complicated social services system, connecting a client to community resources: food banks, child care, education, employment, and much more (Tuohy, 2017). Additionally, they may also be able to extend an invitation to a home group that that they may frequent or other types of group support.

Staffing-wise, peers can greatly assist an interdisciplinary clinical team that may be challenged by larger caseloads and limited opportunities for contact with clients.

Community Support

Community-based self-help
A larger community may also have a local chapter of self-help organizations. These may consist of AA (Alcoholics Anonymous), NA (Narcotics Anonymous), meetings for a particular substance of use (e.g., Cocaine Anonymous), methadone-specific (Methadone Anonymous), or adjunctive meetings for other challenge areas (e.g., Co-Dependents Anonymous).

Anecdotally, a stressor that routinely presents itself to individuals undergoing methadone maintenance is feeling stigmatized by some members from outside self-help meetings. This is because of the controversy associated with replacement therapy and debate over the concept of "being clean."

As such, disclosure of methadone maintenance status and stigma management might be a topic in individual, couple's, and family counseling. Ensuring that a client explores both the advantages and disadvantages associated with possible reactions from their social support network might be something to anticipate. Then, if a client has a sponsor from their home group, it might be beneficial to work in tandem for coordinating community support (activities for relapse prevention, mentorship, and follow-ups) into the participant's treatment, pending both parties' interest.

Self-help organizations such as Narcotics Anonymous do not officially take a stance on MMT clients attending meetings (Narcotics Anonymous World Services, 1996). Feelings associated with themes of "not belonging" or alienation are important to process in therapeutic work; identifying sober social support in accordance with client autonomy is crucial.

Intensive Case Management (ICM) services

Depending on where you are practicing, there might be intensive case management services offered in your area. With an underlying goal of promoting self-sufficiency, case managers are in the community with clients. Services might include helping with housing, employment, or transportation to essential appointments.

Since we are often grounded in one location when serving participants, intensive case managers give a crucial service in accompanying them to appointments within the community. This can be an integral bridge within what we do for a limited amount of time in the treatment facility, and when clients face greater obstacles outside of this space.

Literature surrounding intensive case management services for those suffering from chemical dependency has demonstrated increased treatment retention for outpatient (Rosenblum, Nuttbrock, McQuistion, Magura, & Joseph, 2002) and general aftercare services (Siegal, Li, & Rapp, 2002). This is significant, given that individuals participating in these services often have better holistic treatment outcomes compared to those that do not.

Online communities
With increasing access and demand for the internet came the advent of online support through message boards and internal chat services. As with any community-reinforcement approach, screen and ensure that a potential website is appropriate for the participant.

Age, ethnicity, gender, presenting medical challenges, socioeconomic status, and trauma history are considerations to think about when working with a client to determine whether a resource could be viable. If there are geographical or mental health limitations in linking an individual to community-based support groups, referrals to an online support group might be appropriate.

They can be effective; a review of research on online support groups from 2008 found that many groups have been effective in promoting well-being, a sense of control, self-confidence, feelings of more independence, social interactions, and improved feelings (Barak, Boniel-Nissim, & Suler, 2008). Although in-person support groups could be considered a crucial part of holistic recovery, online communities can offer similar benefits to a client who may encounter difficulties with finding something readily available.

As with any referral, it is essential to work collaboratively with the client in determining whether it is a good fit and aligned with their values. For possible online referrals for a participant seeking additional support, please see the "Useful Websites" section.

Summary

Support comes in many forms, whether it is within the treatment setting itself, out in the larger community, or even online. For many maintaining their sobriety following an inpatient stay, it is difficult to change the "people, places, and things" that are often associated with prior substance use. Moreover, it can take a team of individuals to help overhaul the demands placed on a client when they leave their treatment facility and go back out into the community.

When participants are helped by different agencies of change, altering these former associations can be possible. As with any treatment recommendation, it is equally necessary to work with the client sitting in front of us and meet them where they are.

10: Spirituality

> *"What lies behind us and what lies before us are tiny matters compared to what lies within us."*
> – Ralph Waldo Emerson

The term 'spirituality' has been confused with 'religion.' Now, we often hear the phrase, "I'm not religious, I'm spiritual." Differences between the two terms are significant and can often elicit different reactions from clients. Literature suggests that an understanding of spirituality often includes references to a connection or a relationship with a higher power, which may combine values and beliefs in daily behaviors (Hill et al., 2000).

At a biological level, methadone serves as an effective "silver bullet" for correctively treating the physical withdrawal and certain aspects of the psychological compulsion related with illicit opioid dependence. While a portion of relapse prevention therapy is dedicated to learning how to create a balanced lifestyle more globally (Parks & Marlatt, 2000), working with a client to draw out a deeper spiritual capacity can lay the groundwork for more coping skills for when thoughts to resume use arise. Many experts in addiction agree that utilizing spirituality within a bio-psycho-social-spiritual perspective can be useful in treatment (CAST, 2004a).

"A Spiritual Awakening"

You may have heard of the phrase, "a spiritual awakening." This can often conjure up many images of sudden and radical transformation. However, this "spiritual awakening" may not be as grandiose or eye opening as a person might expect.

For those in recovery, such an awakening can be viewed as a new conscious awareness and state of being. It can be the breaking away from the obsessive, compulsive, and self-centered facets of addiction, and garnering a desire to experience something greater in life. Additionally, there is evidence to suggest that most clients think that spirituality is a positive element to bring into their treatment (Arnold, Avants, Margolin, & Marcotte, 2002).

Bridging Spirituality with Mental Health Counseling

A mental health provider's treatment orientation may include elements of helping a client identify and make sense of their own spiritual beliefs and practices. Third-wave behavior therapies, such as acceptance & commitment therapy (ACT), have offered a window to perform values-explorations and integrate spirituality into the holistic recovery process (Wilson & Murrell, 2004).

Such therapies have a dedicated practice of clinical mindfulness, which is described as "paying attention in a particular way: on purpose, in the present, and nonjudgmentally" (Kabat-Zinn, 2009). Unless you have a dedicated personal practice and the training necessary to teach, it could help to refer a client out to a Mindfulness-Based Stress Reduction (MBSR) course or a mental health provider able to provide this core skillset.

Besides this, journaling, bibliotherapy, and regular self-reflection within the holistic recovery process might be an aspect that could be beneficial in working with a client as well. As with any treatment modality, a participant must be agreeable to it and the practice needs to be aligned with their values.

Spirituality and Self-Help Groups

As discussed in Chapter 9, self-help can be a viable option for providing both community support and spiritual growth in the holistic recovery process. Many popular models stress the reliance on a higher power to help restore an individual to sound mental health following the recognition they are powerless over their substance of choice.

Galanter (2007) describes these social communities as a mechanism that can promote new and transcendent meaning in the lives of those recovering. By ushering in spiritual growth, a client aligned with their values and beliefs can have more resources to help change their behaviors.

It is also important to mention that self-help is not the be-all and end-all to treating addiction, and some clients may not identify this as a significant part of their treatment. That is okay. Given that everyone has been through many different life experiences, there is not a "one size fits all" treatment approach that can effectively manage all substance use issues.

Support from Religious Communities

Besides psychotherapy and self-help groups, a client may also seek guidance from a religious leader in their community to help incorporate this possible aspect of treatment. If treatment allows for it, networking inclusion with a member from the community could be beneficial with better understanding how their religious beliefs can be a part of the spiritual strand of their recovery.

Ultimately, a client is the author of their recovery, and eliciting and maintaining their sobriety may draw from many sources to help foster their spirituality.

Summary

Spirituality is a connection with a higher power that may influence a person's daily behaviors, along with a value or belief system. If adopting a bio-psycho-social-spiritual model in treating addiction, it is essential to consider how spirituality can be fostered within a client's recovery process, as this could be a critical aspect of sustainable behavioral change.

Several ways to develop this with clients could be through the counselor's treatment modalities, self-help model, or connection with religious communities in a client's area. As with any approach, it is important to work within your professional competency and collaboratively with a participant.

11: Nutrition and Exercise
Meghan Morley, LPC, Certified Personal Trainer, Certified Group Fitness Instructor

It is no secret that the key to a healthy life is a balanced wellness plan that includes a sensible diet and regular physical activity. For people in active addiction, these practices are often lost in the drug seeking chaos that consumes their daily lives. Research shows that individuals who are methadone maintained or otherwise exposed to μ-opioid agonists, often experience significant weight gain and are at a higher risk for chronic illnesses related to a lack of physical wellness (Mohs, Wayson, & Leonard-Green, 1990; Nolan & Scagnelli, 2007; Rajs, Thiblin, Olsson-Mortlock, Fredriksson, & Eksborg, 2004). As these individuals make their transition into recovery, it is essential to educate them on how to take care of their bodies, just as much as their minds.

In this chapter, we will explore ways to help educate our clients on the importance of holistic wellness. With person-centered care and respecting our clients' autonomy, it is best practice to communicate through Motivational Interviewing and ask permission before providing the client with educational information (Miller & Rollnick, 2013). Finally, as you apply this information in your sessions, remember the confines of your professional expertise. Unless you are a registered dietitian, personal trainer, or otherwise credentialed professional, you should not be recommending specific diets, meal plans or exercise programming. However, you can educate your clients on healthy eating and activity habits.

Nutrition

Opioid-dependent individuals often have poor nutritional status, low energy level, and a high sugar intake (Zador, Wall, & Webster, 1996). Qualitative inquiries have also found those that are methadone maintained, ingest many snacks and sweets as compared with controls, which results in a higher average BMI - leaving these individuals more susceptible to a number of chronic illnesses (Nolan & Scagelli, 2007). Cookies, cakes, sodas, and high sugar juice products are the preferred snacks for participants in group counseling sessions we have facilitated.

The best approach when aiding our participants with having balanced eating habits is to keep it simple and provide them with useful information that is also culturally and socioeconomically responsive. We want those we serve to understand the importance of regular meals, rather than snacking throughout the day. These meals should comprise a variety of foods that are nutritious and consumed in an appropriate amount. Send a message surrounding the importance of eating a variety of foods from each food group: fruits, vegetables, grains, protein foods and dairy (Choose MyPlate, 2018d). It is important to not assume that participants know examples of foods in each category and to go over them.

The following is an overview of some of the most important messages to get across to clients:

- Encourage your participants to **eat whole foods** in lieu of pre-packaged food. Note the frozen fruits and vegetables are just

as nutritious as fresh and can be a great option when considering cost and food waste concerns.
- Educate clients on the difference between **whole grains**, which have a higher level of vitamin B, fiber, and iron, than refined grains. Additionally, MMT participants will also be interested to know that consuming whole grains can reduce opioid-induced constipation and aid in weight management. Encourage clients to have at least 50% of their consumed grains to be whole grain, including brown rice, whole wheat bread, oatmeal, etc. (Choose MyPlate, 2017b).
- **Protein** is an essential component of nutrition, serving as the building blocks for blood, muscles, skin, bones, hormones, vitamins and enzymes (Choose MyPlate, 2017c). Participants may lack education on the true range of high protein foods, including meat and poultry, eggs, seafood, beans, nuts, soy products, seeds, and peas. Protein is also a key component to weight management, aiding individuals in feeling fuller longer, curbing cravings for snacks, increasing muscle development, and supporting a healthy metabolism and weight loss.
- **Dairy** has a lot of value in terms of sufficient calcium, potassium, vitamin D and protein found in these products. Encourage clients to consume milk, yogurt, and cheese regularly and make known options for alternative non-lactose products for those with sensitivities (Choose MyPlate, 2017a). It is a common myth that methadone rots teeth and makes bones brittle, among other misconceptions. Speak to participants about how their lack of dairy intake may be the

reason for these issues, rather than a side-effect of methadone. For more information, please see the "Common Myths & Facts About MMT" section.

- **Portion control and moderation** are hot-button words in weight management and healthy eating; however, this becomes highly subjective and restraint can be a challenge for anyone, notwithstanding, an individual with a history of impulse control deficits. The U.S. Department of Agriculture suggests women and men over the age of 19 need 1.5-2 cups of fruit per day, 2.5-3 cups of vegetables per day, 5-6.5 oz of protein, 3-4 oz of grains, 3 cups of dairy, and 5-7 teaspoons of oil (Choose MyPlate, 2018a).

- All individuals need a different number of **calories** depending on age, height, weight, activity level and other individual factors. If tracking calories is of interest to the client, there are a number of apps that can be convenient and helpful in logging food. When focusing more on hitting all the major food groups for a balanced diet, the MyPlate Daily Checklist is a simple printable format that is easy to follow (Choose MyPlate, 2018a). Again, remember the limits of your professional knowledge and if necessary, refer participants to a nutritionist or dietician for a more specific meal and dietary planning.

- It may be more accessible, however, to speak more about **plate composition** than in measurements, which can be confusing and bulky. The MyPlate tool is an excellent visual aid to demonstrate the variety and number of good groups needed every meal. As a therapist, you can go on to this website and print out visual aids, quizzes, articles and other interactive content that can be used in session or as homework to engage in for psychoeducation.

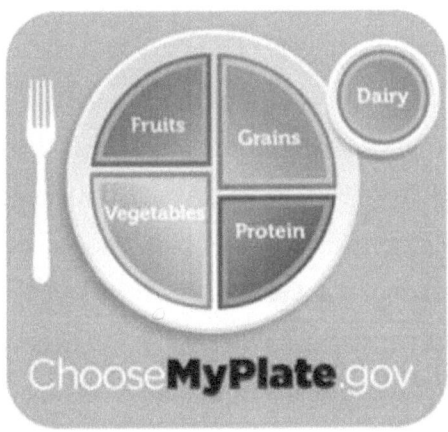

Figure 9. A visual of *MyPlate* and the 5 food groups
www.ChooseMyPlate.gov

Most of the work we do with clients should be focused on healthy foods to eat, rather than a message of deprivation. However, there are a few areas where a message of limiting intake is essential to maintain a healthy diet. Before even introducing these items, it is first helpful to discuss the importance of and how to read a nutrition label with clients. For an excellent tutorial on nutrition labels go to https://www.fda.gov/Food/LabelingNutrition.

- The first product for limitation is **sodium.** It is extremely high in pre-packaged, canned and processed foods; additionally, restaurant and takeout food are also high in sodium. Too much salt can lead to high blood pressure, a condition already common among those taking methadone (O'Toole, Hambly, Cox, O'Shea & Darker, 2014).

- **Fat** is another area to limit, but only trans and saturated fats. Limiting trans and saturated fats can decrease risk for heart disease and increased "bad" cholesterol (Choose MyPlate, 2017d). These fats are found in foods, such as animal fats, butter, whole milk and hydrogenated oils. Instead, urge patients to opt for unsaturated fats found in olive oil, avocado, nuts, seeds, and fish (Choose MyPlate, 2016). Suggest that participants cook with olive oil over butter, drink fat-free or low-fat milk instead of whole milk, choose leaner meats and fish, and eat low-fat cheeses and yogurts.
- Suggest limiting **sugar** intake. Many foods have high levels of naturally occurring sugar, such as fruit, dairy products, and vegetables. These are not the foods we want to tell participants to dial back on; it is added sugars that we want to steer our clients from eating. These sugars are an easy way to blow our recommended calorie intake and lead to weight gain. Speak about limiting intake of baked goods, such as cookies and brownies, candy, jams, syrups and ice cream. Many clients do not understand how much sugar they are consuming through soda, sugary juices, and coffee. Inform participants on how much sugar they are adding to their coffee and how they can taper that amount to decrease their daily sugar intake.

This leads me to my final point, which should be our number one priority in helping clients live a healthier life. Water consumption is essential to all bodily functions and should be the primary beverage consumed (Choose MyPlate, 2018c). Sufficient water intake is associated with removing waste from the body through urination, sweating and bowel movements, as well as regulating body temperature and keeping joints lubricated.

Roughly speaking, humans should be consuming 64 oz of water per day or eight times 8 oz glasses of water (Mayo Clinic, 2017). Water needs vary by individual based on many factors. Increased exercise and a hot or humid environment can mean that an individual needs more water, while other health factors and pregnancy can also mean changes in your fluid needs. Speak to clients about staying ahead of thirst and using the color of their urine to gauge hydration, as urine should be colorless or light yellow.

When educating patients on nutrition, do not leave your counseling skills at the door. This behavioral change is not all that different from the process of ceasing drug use. Use Motivational Interviewing, CBT skills, contingency management and other evidence-based practices to aid the participant in putting these changes into effect. Remember to help patients set clear SMART goals (see *MindTools* in the "Useful Websites" section for more info on how to write these). Most importantly, help patients focus on small changes to build self-efficacy and increase motivation.

Exercise

Exercise is something that America, in general, does not get enough of. Among the general population, almost half of Americans meet the minimum weekly physical activity recommendations. In a study by Caviness, Bird, Anderson, Abrantes, and Stein (2013), only 38% of methadone-maintained individuals met the weekly requirement and nearly a quarter reported no moderate or vigorous physical activity. Exercise as an adjunctive service for individuals in substance abuse treatment has also been shown to increase social engagement, emotional regulation, and stress management, and decrease anxiety sensitivity (Correia, Benson, Carey, 2005). Plus, it is beneficial for reducing the risk of high blood pressure, high blood cholesterol, stroke, type 2 diabetes and heart disease.

The U.S. Department of Health & Human Services (DHHS) suggests that the average adult should get at least 150 minutes per week of moderate-intensity aerobic physical activity for at least 10 minutes at a time and engage in strength-training activities at least two days per week (CDC, 2018). The DHHS website also offers a list of exercise suggestions that can be provided to our clients, which includes going on walks with the family, as well as dancing and swimming at the local recreation center. Medicaid and Medicare recipients are also eligible for membership discounts at local YMCAs and other facilities if they inquire, some as low as $1 per month.

It is also important to be mindful that our clients perceive themselves to be unwell compared to the general population (Millson et al., 2004). As a result, they may be apprehensive to engage in exercise for a number of emotional or physical reasons, which makes the use of Motivational Interviewing an essential component to building their motivation and feelings surrounding self-efficacy (Miller & Rollnick, 2013).

I find it essential to remind my patients that exercise can be simple and done anywhere. Encourage clients to go outside for a walk, look online for free exercise videos, and/or show them the DHHS website for exercise suggestions and information. Additionally, we can also point out that exercise and fitness goals need not be about weight or physical appearance change.

Summary

Promoting a healthy lifestyle through proper nutrition and exercise does not have to be cumbersome. Help patients develop fun and exciting SMART goals, such as completing a physical feat, health-based improvements, and enhancement in mood or other mental health related outcomes. Integrating nutrition and fitness psychoeducation into treatment can support clients with embracing a holistic rooted approach to recovery.

Common Myths and Facts About MMT

Myth: "Methadone rots your teeth and bones."
Fact: Diffuse bone and joint pain can be an indicator of opioid withdrawal (Wesson & Ling, 2003). A client complaining of this discomfort could benefit from having their dose evaluated and possibly adjusted by your program physician.

Myth: "Methadone is toxic and taking it for too long can't be good for you."
Fact: Like with any medication, methadone has a number of observable side effects that are covered in Chapter 4. Since methadone is metabolized in the liver, research has been conducted on liver function in those that have engaged with long-term MMT; damage is often attributed to hepatitis or alcohol use and not the methadone itself (Kreek, Dodes, Kane, Knobler, & Martin, 1972).

Myth: "Methadone is harder to get off of than *dope*."
Fact: As previously discussed in Chapter 1, methadone does stay in the body longer than illicit opioids, which is also the reason why it is so effective in curbing withdrawal symptoms and cravings. As long as a methadone taper is being appropriately supervised by the program physician as well as done in a way that is considerate of a speed, amount, and progress in treatment, a participant can successfully detox from methadone with limited discomfort.

Myth: "Methadone makes people pick up a *coke* or *benzo* habit."

Fact: Even with the use of a corrective medication to counteract opioid withdrawal and physical craving, a person who is still working on finding the lifestyle changes necessary to reduce and abstain from drugs will undoubtedly continue to use substances. Availability of different types of illicit substances where a client lives, works, and plays, may dictate what people are using. They may have even been using these substances prior to starting MMT.

Myth: "Methadone causes people to *nod*."

Fact: If a client is being prescribed an appropriate dosage of methadone to both stop their illicit opioid use as well as cravings, they are undetectable. In fact, you may have unknowingly shared the bus or train today with someone participating in MMT. Concurrent substance use (typically benzodiazepines or illicit opioids) could account for someone dozing off. Also, pre-existing medical conditions may also contribute to their presentation.

Myth: "A low dose of methadone is better for you."

Fact: As mentioned in Chapter 1, most clients are stabilized with 80mg to 120mg of methadone (Joseph, Stancliff, & Langrod, 2000; Mallinckrodt Pharmaceuticals Inc., 2008; Vocci, Acri, & Elkashef, 2005). This therapeutic dosage (which will include outliers depending on clients' body chemistry) is necessary for stopping withdrawal symptoms and mitigating cravings for opioids. A lower dosage has the possibility of supplementing continued illicit opioid use, and not serving its intended purpose in MMT.

Useful Websites

18percent

https://18percent.org/

This is an online support group for those with mental health challenges in addition to substance use. It uses a messaging application called *Slack*, which connects people anonymously plus provides support and community.

After Silence

http://www.aftersilence.org/

"An online support group, message board, and chat room for rape, sexual assault, and sexual abuse survivors." Offers these means to receive additional support, as well as resources of all formats for recovering from rape and sexual abuse.

Al-Anon

https://al-anon.org/al-anon-meetings/find-an-al-anon-meeting/

This is a website that gives meeting locations for those wanting support when they have someone in their life challenged by a drinking problem.

Alcoholics Anonymous (AA)

https://www.aa.org/pages/en_US/find-local-aa

Website that gives information on how to find local AA chapters within a specific area.

The American Association of Sexuality Educators, Counselors and Therapists (AASECT)

https://www.aasect.org/

AASECT is a non-profit organization that is dedicated to bringing together professionals that are involved in promoting the understanding of human sexuality and healthy human behavior. Along with offering certifications as a sexuality educator, sexuality counselor, sex therapist and supervisor, they also give information surrounding continuing education in this nuanced treatment population.

The American Association for the Treatment of Opioid Dependence (AATOD)

http://www.aatod.org/

Organization dedicated to enhancing the quality of care in treatment programs by promoting the growth and development of comprehensive opioid treatment services throughout the United States. Hosts projects and educational trainings on advancing the field of medication-assisted treatment.

Cocaine Anonymous (CA)

https://ca.org/meetings/

This is a link to online information for individuals that may be challenged by concurrent cocaine addiction who want community and support through a local chapter of CA.

Co-Dependents Anonymous (CoDA)

http://locator.coda.org/

The above web address can be a useful resource for those that are struggling with co-dependency in their holistic recovery efforts.

Crisis Text Line

https://www.crisistextline.org/

Crisis Text Line is an electronic platform that allows anyone in the U.S. to text "HOME" to 741741 and connect with a live crisis counselor to help them work through painful emotions. Crisis counselors work with anonymous texters to help bring them from a "hot moment" to a "calm cool," as well as assess for suicidality.

Crystal Meth Anonymous (CMA)

https://crystalmeth.org/cma-meetings/meeting-search.html

Website that has searchable map of support groups for those challenged by methamphetamine dependency.

The Drug Policy Alliance

http://www.drugpolicy.org/

A broad coalition of organizations aimed at advancing "those policies and attitudes that best reduce the harms of both drug use and drug prohibition, and to promote the sovereignty of individuals over their minds and bodies." DPA publishes work for consumers on harm reduction and methadone maintenance.

Harm Reduction Coalition

http://harmreduction.org/

A diverse network of allies who are working towards challenging the stigma faced by people who use drugs (PWUDs) while also advocating for policy and public health reform. Harm Reduction Coalition disseminates resources on overdose prevention, hepatitis C, and information on tools used to reduce harm with PWUDs.

Huddle
https://hihuddle.com/

An application for those with smartphones that allows users to join messaging groups focused in mental health topics, such as: addiction, body positivity, depression, and stress & anxiety.

Inspire
https://www.inspire.com/

Online messaging forum for those that have been affected by co-occurring health conditions. Inspire strives to connect patients and caregivers to health information and support.

Legal Action Center
https://lac.org/

Non-profit organization dedicated to "fight discrimination against people with histories of addiction, HIV/AIDS, or criminal records, and to advocate for sound public policies in these areas." LAC houses information and sample letters on advocacy for individuals challenged by discrimination due to their status.

Marijuana Anonymous (MA)
https://www.marijuana-anonymous.org/meetings/find

This is a link for participants interested in locating a local chapter of Marijuana Anonymous for fellowship and support.

Methadone.us
http://www.methadone.us/methadone-clinics/

A collaborative that hosts information on methadone programs around the United States. In addition to contact information for Medicaid-funded programs, there is also a list of physicians eligible to prescribe methadone.

MindTools
https://www.mindtools.com/

Offers an online toolkit on decision making, interpersonal skills, and problem solving that is relevant for clinicians. Also gives a thorough breakdown of SMART goals.

NAADAC, the Association for Addiction Professionals
https://www.naadac.org/

Professional organization dedicated to providing education, certification, and clinical training to those treating addiction. Members are offered 145 hours of free continuing education through online webinars.

Nar-Anon
https://www.nar-anon.org/find-a-meeting/

This is a website that helps families and friends of those with addiction find a self-help group for additional community and support.

National Institute on Drug Abuse (NIDA)
https://www.drugabuse.gov/

Part of the United States Department of Health and Human Services that is focused specifically on the science associated with substance use. Their website offers a collection of statistics on current drug trends, as well as general information on substances of abuse.

Narcotics Anonymous (NA)
https://www.na.org/meetingsearch/

Website that gives information on how to find local NA chapters within a searchable area.

National Alliance for Medication Assisted Treatment (NAMA)
http://www.methadone.org/

NAMA is a union of "patients, healthcare professionals, friends, and associates working together for greater public understanding and acceptance of MAT." Along with advocacy, information on MMT, and efforts to de-stigmatize, NAMA also hosts a MAT Advocate Certification Committee that oversees the Certified Medication Assisted Treatment (MAT) Advocate (CMA) credential.

National Alliance on Mental Illness (NAMI)
https://www.nami.org/

NAMI is a mental health organization that is intended to provide education, advocacy for public policy, a lifeline for those that need help, and public awareness events and activities.

The National Center for PTSD
https://www.ptsd.va.gov/index.asp

Agency within the U.S. Department of Veterans Affairs that is dedicated to the research and education of trauma and PTSD. Houses information on screening, assessment tools, and types of evidence-based treatment available.

The National Domestic Violence Hotline
https://www.thehotline.org/

Hotline (800-799-7233) and confidential chatroom offering 24/7 confidential immediate support to enable victims to find tools to "live lives free of abuse." Also gives information to visitors about what abuse and healthy relationships look like. The website has numerous resources for victims and survivors.

The National Suicide Prevention Lifeline
https://suicidepreventionlifeline.org/

A 24/7 number (800-273-8255) that provides free confidential support for those that have found themselves in distress, whether it means prevention or crisis management. Along with this, the National Suicide Prevention Lifeline also gives best practices information to providers on suicide risk assessment standards.

Overeaters Anonymous (OA)
https://oa.org/find-a-meeting/

This resource provides a link to OA meetings in an area. They offer support for those challenged by "compulsive overeating, under-eating, food addiction, anorexia, bulimia, binge eating, or overexercising."

Psychology Tools
https://www.psychologytools.com/

Houses a bank of different print outs for clients, subdivided into problem areas, treatment orientations, techniques, and mechanisms of action. Trials allow for 5 free worksheet downloads.

Rape, Abuse & Incest National Network (RAINN)
https://www.rainn.org/

RAINN has a 24/7 hotline (800-656-4673) plus live chat for those seeking confidential support in surviving sexual violence. Additionally, this organization offers services for victims, public education, advocacy for laws and regulations to improve public policy, as well as consultation and training.

The Substance Abuse and Mental Health Services Administration (SAMHSA)

https://www.samhsa.gov/

Agency within the U.S. Department of Health and Human Services that offers information, services, and research surrounding substance use. Agencies can also order free publications that help both clinicians and consumers in delivering and receiving competent treatment.

The Travel Resource Center

https://indro-online.de/en/methadone-worldwide-travel-guide/

This is a travel guide index that gives information on the status of methadone maintenance treatment in a country, whether importation of methadone is possible, and ways to get more facts from the host location.

The Trevor Project

https://www.thetrevorproject.org/

An organization dedicated to providing crisis intervention and suicide prevention services to lesbian, gay, bisexual, transgender, queer & questioning individuals under the age of 25. In addition to programs for youth, Trevor Project also offers training and resources for both professionals and advocates.

Useful Books

Bisaga, A. (2018). *Overcoming opioid addiction: The authoritative medical guide for patients, families, doctors, and therapists.* The Experiment.

Foote, J., Wilkens, C., Kosanke, N., & Higgs, S. (2014). *Beyond addiction: How science and kindness help people change.* Simon and Schuster.

Hari, J. (2016). *Chasing the scream: The first and last days of the war on drugs.* Bloomsbury USA.

Herman, J. L. (2015). *Trauma and recovery: The aftermath of violence—from domestic abuse to political terror.* Basic Books.

Janes, R. (2010). *Methadone: Bad boy of drug treatment: What works & what doesn't.* Outskirts Press, Incorporated.

Kuhar, M. (2011). *The addicted brain: Why we abuse drugs, alcohol, and nicotine.* FT Press.

Maté, G. (2010). *In the realm of hungry ghosts: Close encounters with addiction.* North Atlantic Books.

Perry, B. D., & Szalavitz, M. (2017). *The boy who was raised as a dog: And other stories from a child psychiatrist's notebook—what traumatized children can teach us about loss, love, and healing.* Basic Books.

Szalavitz, M. (2016). *Unbroken brain: a revolutionary new way of understanding addiction.* St. Martin's Press.

Thomas, P. & Margulis, J. (2016). *The addiction spectrum: A compassionate, holistic approach to recovery.* HarperOne.

Glossary*

#

420: (*n.*) can refer to April 20th, a holiday celebrating marijuana counterculture.

A

Abscess: (*n.*) a confined pocket of pus typically from infection via intravenous drug usage.
Acid: (*n.*) referring to lysergic acid (LSD).
Angel dust: (*n.*) PCP in powdered form. Also available in tablets and oil.

B

Bar: (n.) a 2mg tablet of Xanax® that resembles a rectangular bar.
Bake: (*v.*) to smoke marijuana.
Bang: (*v.*) to use a substance intravenously.
Benzo: (*n.*) refers to the benzodiazepine psychoactive drug class.
Biscuit: (*n.*) a 40mg tablet of methadone that has been largely replaced by liquid methadone.
Black tar heroin: (*n.*) heroin that is black and sticky in appearance and needs to be prepared before use. Often found in Western and Southern parts of the United States.

Blocker: (*n.*) a methadone dosage that is marked by an abstinence from illicit opioids and lack of withdrawal symptoms.

Blow: (*n.*) cocaine. Also referred to as *coke* or *powder*.

Blunt: (*n.*) a cigar that is hollowed out and filled with marijuana to be smoked.

Boost: (*v.*) to shoplift.

Box: (*n.*) a lockbox used to store take-home dosages.

Brick: (*n.*) a collection of 5 *bundles* of heroin, or around 50 bags of heroin in total.

Bud: (*n.*) marijuana. Also referred to as *dope, grass,* or *weed*.

Bundle: (*n.*) typically 8-10 bags of heroin wrapped in a rubber band and distributed.

C

Cap: (*n.*) the top of a psychedelic mushroom.

Catty: (*n.*) short for Catapres® or clonidine. This anti-hypertensive is contraindicated with methadone.

China White: (*n.*) an analog of heroin that is typically laced with fentanyl or carfentanil. It is most often found in the Eastern United States.

Cop: (*v.*) to purchase illicit substances often through questionable means.

Crank: (*n.*) methamphetamine. Also referred to as *speed*.

Crib: (*n.*) where a person lives.

Cut: (*v.*) to dilute a drug with another potentially undesirable substance.

D

Dab: 1. (*n.*) THC extract.

    2. (v.) a dance move possibly originating from the sneezing associated with smoking a large amount of cannabis.

Dank: (*adj.*) used to describe something of good quality, typically marijuana.

DHS: (*n., abr.*) Department of Human Services.

Dime bag: (*n.*) a $10 bag of a substance.

Dipper: (*n.*) a cigarette that is dipped in phencyclidine oil.

Dolly: (*n.*) a Dolophine® methadone tablet.

Dope: 1. (*n.*) heroin

    2. (*n.*) refers to marijuana in certain regions.

    3. (*adj.*) used to describe something as cool, nice, or awesome.

Dope man: (*n.*) a drug dealer that distributes heroin.

E

Edible: (*n.*) any edible product containing THC.

F

Flakka: (*n.*) a type of bath salt.

Football: (*n.*) a 1mg tablet of Xanax® that takes the appearance of a prolate spheroid.

Forty: (*n.*) a 40oz. bottle of malt liquor or beer.

G

GHB: (*n., abr.*) short for *gamma*-Hydroxybutyric acid. This is commonly known to the public as a date-rape drug and anesthetic used to treat narcolepsy.

Grass: (*n.*) marijuana. Also referred to as *bud, dope,* or *weed.*

H

Hard: (*n.*) crack cocaine.

Hash: (*n.*) a concentrated form of the chemical THC (in marijuana) that is available in oil and hard resin forms.

Huff: (*v.*) to intentionally inhale fumes.

I

Ice: (*n.*) methamphetamine. Also referred to as *crank,* or *speed.*

J

Joint: (*n.*) a cigarette that is rolled with marijuana.

Juice: 1. (*n.*) methadone.
   2. (*n.*) e-cigarette fluid.

K

K2: (*n.*) synthetic cannabinoid. Also referred to as *spice.*

L

Lace: (*v.*) to add one substance to another.

Lean: (*n.*) a narcotic beverage concocted from promethazine, codeine cough syrup and lemon-lime soft drink.
Loosey: (*n.*) a single cigarette.
LSD: (*n., abr.*) lysergic acid.

M

Molly: (*n.*) an allegedly pure form of MDMA (ecstasy) that is in capsule and powder forms.

N

Nickel bag: (*n.*) a $5 bag of a substance.
Nod: (*v.*) to doze off when intoxicated with opioids.

O

Oxy: (*n.*) Oxycodone.

P

PCP: (*n., abr.*) short for phencyclidine, a dissociative drug.
Peach: (*n.*) a .5mg tablet of Klonopin®.
Perc: (*n.*) short for Percocet®.
Piece: (*n.*) a firearm.
Pin: (*n.*) short for Klonopin®.
Powder: (*n.*) cocaine. Also referred to as "blow," or "coke."

R

Rock: (*n.*) a crack rock.

Roids: (*n.*) anabolic steroids.

Roll: (*v.*) to experience an ecstasy trip.

S

Sample: (*n.*) a bag of heroin that is distributed for free to users. The purpose of this is to gauge the purity. Also called a *tester*.

Shoot: (*v.*) to use a substance intravenously. Also referred to as *banging* in certain regions.

Skitz: (*v.*) to undergo self-induced psychosis through substance use, typically from stimulants.

Smack: (*n.*) heroin. Also referred to as *dope*.

Special K: (*n.*) ketamine.

Speed: (*n.*) amphetamine. Also referred to as *crank*.

Speedball: (*n.*) a combination of heroin and cocaine.

Spice: (*n.*) synthetic cannabinoid. Also referred to as *K2*.

Spliff: (*n.*) a cone-shaped cigarette rolled with marijuana.

Stack: (*n.*) $1000.

Stamp: (*n.*) a brand used by drug dealers that is placed on the glassine heroin bag. See Fig. 2.

Stash: 1. (*n.*) a place where illicit substances or money are put away. 2. (*v.*) to hide illicit substances or money.

Stem: (*n.*) a glass pipe often purchased at gas stations to smoke crack cocaine.

Straight shooter: (*n.*) a crack pipe.

Straw: (*n.*) tube used to inhale powdered substances.

Subs: (*n.*) short for Suboxone®.

Syrup: (*n.*) promethazine with codeine.

T

T: (*n.*) a capital letter that refers to methamphetamine.

Take-home: (*n.*) a prescribed dosage of methadone that a client can take back to their residence, limiting contact with their clinic.

Teena: (*n.*) a bag of methamphetamine that is typically sold in 1/16th oz.

Tester: (*n.*) a bag of heroin that is distributed to users for free. The purpose of this is to gauge the purity. Also known as a *sample*.

THC: (*n., abr.*) short for Tetrahydrocannabinol, the active ingredient in marijuana.

Toke: (*v.*) to inhale marijuana.

Track mark: (*n.*) a hole or scar from injecting substances intravenously.

Traphouse: (*n.*) a house where drugs are sold, typically located in an impoverished neighborhood.

Trick: 1. (*n.*) a prostitute.
   2. (*v.*) to engage in prostitution.

Turbo: (*n.*) a combination of marijuana and cocaine that is typically rolled up in a cigarette and smoked.

Tweak: (*v.*) to be under the influence of amphetamines and engage in bizarre behavior.

W

Weed: (*n.*) marijuana. Also referred to as *bud, dope,* or *grass*.

Wet: (*n.*) phencyclidine in oil form.

Whippet: (*n.*) pressurized nitrous oxide in a can of whipped cream.

Works: (*n.*) needles and other drug paraphernalia used to inject substances.

X

X: (*n.*) ecstacy.
Xanny: (*n.*) Xanax®.

*This is not an exhaustive list of terminology in the methadone maintenance community and may also vary with the region that you are serving in.

References

ACOG Committee on Health Care for Underserved Women. (2012). ACOG Committee Opinion No. 524: Opioid abuse, dependence, and addiction in pregnancy. *Obstetrics and gynecology, 119*(5), 1070.

Al-Aawani, A., & Basu, N. (2004). Methadone and excessive sweating. *Addiction, 99*(2), 259-259.

Al-Anon. (2016). *Al-Anon: then & now a brief history* [Brochure]. Virginia Beach, VA: Al-Anon Family Group Headquarters, Inc.

American Psychiatric Association. (2013). *Diagnostic and statistical manual of mental disorders* (5th ed.). Arlington, VA: American Psychiatric Publishing.

Amrhein, P. C., Miller, W. R., Yahne, C. E., Palmer, M., & Fulcher, L. (2003). Client commitment language during motivational interviewing predicts drug use outcomes. *Journal of consulting and clinical psychology, 71*(5), 862

Amrhein, P. C. (2004). How does motivational interviewing work? What client talk reveals. *Journal of Cognitive Psychotherapy, 18*(4), 323-336.

Arnold, R., Avants, S. K., Margolin, A., & Marcotte, D. (2002). Patient attitudes concerning the inclusion of spirituality into addiction treatment. *Journal of substance abuse treatment, 23*(4), 319-326.

Ball, J. C., & Ross, A. (2012). The effectiveness of methadone maintenance treatment: patients, programs, services, and outcome. Springer Science & Business Media.

Barak, A., Boniel-Nissim, M., & Suler, J. (2008). Fostering empowerment in online support groups. *Computers in human behavior, 24*(5), 1867-1883.

Baxter Sr, L. E., Campbell, A., DeShields, M., Levounis, P., Martin, J. A., McNicholas, L., ... & Wilford, B. B. (2013). Safe methadone induction and stabilization: report of an expert panel. *Journal of addiction medicine, 7*(6), 377-386.

Bogucka-Bonikowska, A., Baran-Furga, H., Chmielewska, K., Habrat, B., Scinska, A., Kukwa, A., ... & Bienkowski, P. (2002). Taste function in methadone-maintained opioid-dependent men. *Drug and alcohol dependence, 68*(1), 113-117.

Boisvert, R. A., Martin, L. M., Grosek, M., & Clarie, A. J. (2008). Effectiveness of a peer-support community in addiction recovery: participation as intervention. *Occupational Therapy International, 15*(4), 205-220.

The Bowen Center. (2018). *Eight concepts.* Retrieved from http://thebowencenter.org/theory/eight-concepts/

Brady, K. T., Back, S. E., & Coffey, S. F. (2004). Substance abuse and posttraumatic stress disorder. *Current Directions in Psychological Science, 13*(5), 206-209.

Caruso, Phil (2017, October 24). *Walgreens stocking life saving Narcan® nasal spray in all pharmacies nationwide.* Retrieved from http://news.walgreens.com/press-releases/general-news/walgreens-stocking-life-saving-narcan-nasal-spray-in-all-pharmacies-nationwide.htm

Caflisch, C., Figner, B., & Eich, D. (2003). Biperiden for excessive sweating from methadone. *American Journal of Psychiatry, 160*(2), 386-387.

Caviness, C. M., Bird, J. L., Anderson, B. J., Abrantes, A. M., & Stein, M. D. (2013). Minimum recommended physical activity, and perceived barriers and benefits of exercise in methadone maintained persons. *Journal of Substance Abuse Treatment, 44*(4), 457-462. doi:10.1016/j.jsat.2012.10.002

Center for Evidence-Based Practices. (2010). *Readiness Ruler.* Retrieved from https://www.centerforebp.case.edu/resources/tools/readiness-ruler

Center for Substance Abuse Treatment. (2004a). Chapter 2 impact of substance abuse on families. In *Substance abuse treatment and family therapy.* Rockville, MD: Substance Abuse and Mental Health Services Administration (US).

Center for Substance Abuse Treatment. (2004b). Clinical guidelines for the use of buprenorphine in the treatment of opioid addiction.

Center for Substance Abuse Treatment. (2009). Incorporating alcohol pharmacotherapies into medical practice.

Center for the Treatment and Study of Anxiety (2018a). *About Prolonged Exposure Therapy.* Retrieved from https://www.med.upenn.edu/ctsa/workshops_pet.html

Center for the Treatment and Study of Anxiety (2018b). *Treatment programs at the CTSA.* Retrieved from https://www.med.upenn.edu/ctsa/workshops_pet.html

Centers for Disease Control and Prevention. (2018). *How much physical activity do adults need?* Retrieved from https://www.cdc.gov/physicalactivity/basics/adults/index.htm

Chesher, G. B. (1989). Understanding the opioid analgesics and their effects on skills performance. *Alcohol, drugs and driving, 5*(HS-040 796).

Chey, W. D., Webster, L., Sostek, M., Lappalainen, J., Barker, P. N., & Tack, J. (2014). Naloxegol for opioid-induced constipation in patients with noncancer pain. *New England Journal of Medicine, 370*(25), 2387- 2396.

Choose MyPlate. (2016). *Choosing foods and beverages* Retrieved from https://www.choosemyplate.gov/choosing-foods-and-beverages

Choose MyPlate. (2017a). *All about the dairy group.* Retrieved from https://www.choosemyplate.gov/dairy

Choose MyPlate (2017b). *All about the grains group.* Retrieved from https://www.choosemyplate.gov/grains

Choose MyPlate. (2017c). *All about the protein foods group.* Retrieved from https://www.choosemyplate.gov/protein-foods

Choose MyPlate. (2017d). *Saturated, unsaturated, and trans fats.* Retrieved from https://www.choosemyplate.gov/saturated-unsaturated-and-trans-fats

Choose MyPlate (2018a). *MyPlate plan.* Retrieved from https://www.choosemyplate.gov/MyPlate-Daily-Checklist

Choose MyPlate (2018b). *Other ingredients to consider.* Retrieved from https://www.choosemyplate.gov/other-ingredients-consider

Choose MyPlate. (2018c). *Translating the dietary guidelines into consumer messages.* Retrieved from https://www.choosemyplate.gov/translating-dietary-guidelines-consumer-messages

Choose MyPlate (2018d). *What is MyPlate?* Retrieved from https://www.choosemyplate.gov/MyPlate

Chumpitaz-Corredor, D., & Lara-Solares, A. (2012). Existe correlación entre la dosis de opioide y el tiempo de respuesta a metilnaltrexona [There is a correlation between the dose of opioid and the response time to methylnaltexone]. *Journal of the Spanish Society of Pain,* 19(1), 11-17.

Cnattingius, S. (2004). The epidemiology of smoking during pregnancy: smoking prevalence, maternal characteristics, and pregnancy outcomes. *Nicotine & Tobacco Research: Official Journal of the Society for Research on Nicotine and Tobacco, 6 Suppl 2,* S125-140.

Cognitive Processing Therapy for PTSD (n.d.). *About CPT.* Retrieved from https://cptforptsd.com/about-cpt/

Connock, M., Juarez-Garcia, A., Jowett, S., Frew, E., Liu, Z., Taylor, R. J., ... & Burls, A. (2007). Methadone and buprenorphine for the management of opioid dependence: a systematic review and economic evaluation.

Correia, C. J., Benson, T. A., & Carey, K. B. (2005). Decreased substance use following increases in alternative behaviors: A preliminary investigation. *Addictive Behaviors,30*(1), 19-27. doi:10.1016/j.addbeh.2004.04.006

Cushman, P. (1974). Detoxification of rehabilitated methadone patients: Frequency and predictors of long-term success. *The American journal of drug and alcohol abuse, 1*(3), 393-408.

Darke, S., Larney, S., & Farrell, M. (2017). Yes, people can die from opiate withdrawal. *Addiction, 112*(2), 199-200.

Davis, C. A., Levitan, R. D., Reid, C., Carter, J. C., Kaplan, A. S., Patte, K. A., ... & Kennedy, J. L. (2009). Dopamine for "wanting" and opioids for "liking": a comparison of obese adults with and without binge eating. *Obesity, 17*(6), 1220-1225.

Dick, D. M., & Agrawal, A. (2008). The genetics of alcohol and other drug dependence. *Alcohol Research & Health, 31*(2), 111.

Dolan, K. A., Shearer, J., White, B., Zhou, J., Kaldor, J., & Wodak, A. D. (2005). Four-year follow-up of imprisoned male heroin users and methadone treatment: mortality, re-incarceration and hepatitis C infection. *Addiction, 100*(6), 820-828.

Dunn, K. E., Sigmon, S. C., Reimann, E., Heil, S. H., & Higgins, S. T. (2009). Effects of smoking cessation on illicit drug use among opioid maintenance patients: a pilot study. *Journal of drug issues, 39*(2), 313- 327.

Eidelman, A. I., Schanler, R. J., Johnston, M., Landers, S., Noble, L., Szucs, K., & Viehmann, L. (2012). Breastfeeding and the use of human milk. *Pediatrics, 129*(3), e827-e841.

EMDR Institute, Inc. (2018). *What is EMDR?* Retrieved from http://www.emdr.com/what-is-emdr/

Felitti, V. J., Anda, R. F., Nordenberg, D., Williamson, D. F., Spitz, A. M., Edwards, V., ... & Marks, J. S. (1998). Relationship of childhood abuse and household dysfunction to many of the leading causes of death in adults: The Adverse Childhood Experiences (ACE) Study. *American journal of preventive medicine, 14*(4), 245-258.

Fenn, J. M., Laurent, J. S., & Sigmon, S. C. (2015). Increases in body mass index following initiation of methadone treatment. *Journal of substance abuse treatment, 51,* 59-63.

Feudtner, C., Freedman, J., Kang, T., Womer, J. W., Dai, D., & Faerber, J. (2014). Comparative effectiveness of senna to prevent problematic constipation in pediatric oncology patients receiving opioids: a multicenter study of clinically detailed administrative data. *Journal of pain and symptom management, 48*(2), 272-280.

Frank, J. W., Levy, C., Matlock, D. D., Calcaterra, S. L., Mueller, S. R., Koester, S., & Binswanger, I. A. (2016). Patients' perspectives on tapering of chronic opioid therapy: a qualitative study. *Pain Medicine, 17*(10), 1838-1847.

Gaalema, D. E., Scott, T. L., Heil, S. H., Coyle, M. G., Kaltenbach, K., Badger, G.J., … Jones, H. E. (2012). Differences in the profile of neonatal abstinence syndrome signs in methadone- versus buprenorphine-exposed neonates. *Addiction (Abingdon, England), 107 Suppl 1,* 53–62.

Galanter, M. (2007). Spirituality and recovery in 12-step programs: An empirical model. *Journal of Substance Abuse Treatment, 33*(3), 265-272.

Gutstein, H. B., & Akil, H. (2001). Goodman and Gilman's The Pharmacological Basis of Therapeutics (Hardman JG and Limbird LE eds) pp. 569-619.

Hagan, H., Thiede, H., & Des Jarlais, D. C. (2005). HIV/hepatitis C virus co-infection in drug users: risk behavior and prevention. *AIDS, 19*, S199-S207.

Harm Reduction Coalition. (2018a). *Principles of harm reduction*. Retrieved from https://harmreduction.org/about-us/principles-of-harm-reduction/

Harm Reduction Coalition. (2018b). *Recognizing opioid overdose*. Retrieved from http://harmreduction.org/issues/overdose-prevention/overview/overdose-basics/recognizing-opioid-overdose/

Harm Reduction International (2017). *What is harm reduction?* Retrieved from https://www.hri.global/what-is-harm-reduction

Herman, J. L. (1992). Trauma and recovery. New York, NY, US: Basic Books.

Hill, P. C., Pargament, K. I., Hood, R. W., McCullough Jr, M. E., Swyers, J. P., Larson, D. B., & Zinnbauer, B. J. (2000). Conceptualizing religion and spirituality: Points of commonality, points of departure. *Journal for the theory of social behaviour, 30*(1), 51-77.

Holbrook, A., & Kaltenbach, K. (2012). Co-occurring psychiatric symptoms in opioid-dependent women: the prevalence of antenatal and postnatal depression. *The American Journal of Drug and Alcohol Abuse, 38*(6), 575–579.

Hyland, P., Shevlin, M., Brewin, C. R., Cloitre, M., Downes, A. J., Jumbe, S., ... & Roberts, N. P. (2017). Validation of post-traumatic stress disorder (PTSD) and complex PTSD using the International

Trauma Questionnaire. *Acta Psychiatrica Scandinavica, 136*(3), 313-322.

Indivior Inc. (2018) SUBOXONE® (buprenorphine and naloxone) sublingual film, for sublingual or buccal use CIII (package insert) North Chesterfield, VA: Indivior Inc.

Jones, H. E., Heil, S. H., Tuten, M., Chisolm, M. S., Foster, J. M., O'Grady, K. E., & Kaltenbach, K. (2013). Cigarette smoking in opioid-dependent pregnant women: neonatal and maternal outcomes. *Drug and alcohol dependence, 131*(3), 271-277.

Joseph, H., Stancliff, S., & Langrod, J. (2000). Methadone maintenance treatment (MMT). *The Mount Sinai Journal of Medicine.*

Kabat-Zinn, J. (2009). *Wherever you go, there you are: Mindfulness meditation in everyday life.* Hachette UK.

Kaltenbach, K., Holbrook, A. M., Coyle, M. G., Heil, S. H., Salisbury, A. L., Stine, S. M., … Jones, H. E. (2012). Predicting treatment for neonatal abstinence syndrome in infants born to women maintained on opioid agonist medication. *Addiction (Abingdon, England), 107 Suppl 1*, 45–52.

Kaltenbach, K., O'Grady, K. E., Heil, S. H., Salisbury, A. L., Coyle, M. G., Fischer, G., … Jones, H. E. (2018). Prenatal exposure to methadone or buprenorphine: Early childhood developmental outcomes. *Drug and Alcohol Dependence, 185*, 40–49.

Kampman, K., & Jarvis, M. (2015). American Society of Addiction Medicine (ASAM) National Practice Guideline for the Use of Medications in the Treatment of Addiction Involving Opioid Use. *Journal of Addiction Medicine, 9*(5), 358–367.

Kleber, H. D. (2008). Methadone maintenance 4 decades later. Jama, 300(19), 2303-2305.

Kolarzyk, E., Pach, D., Wojtowicz, B., Szpanowska-Wohn, A., & Szurkowska, M. (2005). Nutritional status of the opiate dependent persons after 4 years of methadone maintenance treatment. *Przeglad lekarski, 62*(6), 373-377.

Kosten, T. R., & George, T. P. (2002). The neurobiology of opioid dependence: implications for treatment. *Science & Practice Perspectives, 1*(1), 13.

Kreek, M. J., Dodes, L., Kane, S., Knobler, J., & Martin, R. (1972). Long- term methadone maintenance therapy: effects on liver function. *Annals of internal medicine, 77*(4), 598-602.

Laudet, A. B., & White, W. L. (2008). Recovery capital as prospective predictor of sustained recovery, life satisfaction, and stress among former poly-substance users. *Substance use & misuse, 43*(1), 27-54.

Leavitt, S. B., Shinderman, M., Maxwell, S., Eap, C. B., & Paris, P. (2000). When "Enough" Is Not Enough. *New perspectives on optimal methadone maintenance dose. The Mount Sinai J. Med, 67*(5-6), 404-11.

Lutz, P. E., & Kieffer, B. L. (2013). The multiple facets of opioid receptor function: implications for addiction. *Current opinion in neurobiology, 23*(4), 473-479.

Mallinckrodt Pharmaceuticals Inc. (2008). Methadose™ Oral Concentrate (methadone hydrochloride oral concentrate USP) and Methadose™ Sugar-Free Oral Concentrate (methadone hydrochloride oral concentrate USP) dye-free, sugar-free, unflavored (package insert). Hazelwood, MO: Mallinckrodt Pharmaceuticals Inc.

Maremmani, I., Pacini, M., Lubrano, S., & Lovrecic, M. (2003). When "enough" is still not "enough": effectiveness of high-dose methadone in the treatment of heroin addiction. *Heroin Add & Rel Clin Probl*, 5(1), 17-32.

Marlatt, G. A., Larimer, M. E., & Witkiewitz, K. (Eds.). (2011). Harm reduction: Pragmatic strategies for managing high-risk behaviors. Guilford Press.

Marsch, L. A. (1998). The efficacy of methadone maintenance interventions in reducing illicit opiate use, HIV risk behavior and criminality: a meta-analysis. Addiction, 93(4), 515-532.

Mattick, R. P., Breen, C., Kimber, J., & Davoli, M. (2009). Methadone maintenance therapy versus no opioid replacement therapy for opioid dependence. *The Cochrane Library*.

Mayo Clinic (2017). *Water: How much should you drink every day?* Retrieved from https://www.mayoclinic.org/healthy-lifestyle/nutrition-and-healthy-eating/in-depth/water/art-20044256

McCance-Katz, E. F., Sullivan, L. E., & Nallani, S. (2010). Drug interactions of clinical importance among the opioids, methadone and buprenorphine, and other frequently prescribed medications: a review. *The American Journal on Addictions*, 19(1), 4-16.

McLellan, A. T., Lewis, D. C., O'brien, C. P., & Kleber, H. D. (2000). Drug dependence, a chronic medical illness: implications for treatment, insurance, and outcomes evaluation. Jama, 284(13), 1689-1695.

Miller, W. R., & Rollnick, S. (2009). Ten things that motivational interviewing is not. *Behavioural and cognitive psychotherapy, 37*(2), 129-140.

Miller, W. R., & Rollnick, S. (2013). Motivational interviewing: helping people change (3rd ed). New York, NY: Guilford Press.

Millson, P.E., Challacombe, L., Villeneuve, P.J., Fischer, B., Strike, C.J., Myers, T., et al. (2004). Self-perceived health among Canadian opiate users: a comparison to the general population and to other chronic disease populations. Canadian Journal of Public Health, 95(2):99–103.

Mohs, M. E., Watson, R. R., & Leonard-Green, T. (1990). Nutritional effects of marijuana, heroin, cocaine, and nicotine. *Journal of the American Dietetic Association, 90,* 1261-1267.

Moolchan, E. T., & Hoffman, J. A. (1994). Phases of treatment: A practical approach to methadone maintenance treatment. *International Journal of the Addictions, 29*(2), 135-160.

Müller-Lissner, S., Bassotti, G., Coffin, B., Drewes, A. M., Breivik, H., Eisenberg, E., ... & Morlion, B. (2017). Opioid-induced constipation and bowel dysfunction: a clinical guideline. *Pain Medicine, 18*(10), 1837- 1863.

Mysels, D. J., & Sullivan, M. A. (2010). The relationship between opioid and sugar intake: review of evidence and clinical applications. *Journal of opioid management, 6*(6), 445.

Narcan® (2017). *More questions?* Retrieved from https://www.narcan.com/faqs

Narcotics Anonymous World Services (1996). *Bulletin #29*. Retrieved from https://www.na.org/?ID=bulletins-bull29

National Archives and Records Administration. (1972) *Federal Register: 37 Fed. Reg. 26701*. Friday. [Periodical] Retrieved from the Library of Congress, https://www.loc.gov/item/fr037242/.

National Center for Health Statistics. (2017). Provisional counts of drug overdose deaths, as of 8/6/2017 (Graph). *Centers for Disease Control*. Retrieved from https://www.cdc.gov/nchs/data/health_policy/monthly-drugoverdose-death-estimates.pdf

National Institute on Drug Abuse. (2018a). *Overdose death rates*. Retrieved from https://www.drugabuse.gov/related-topics/trends-statistics/overdose-death-rates

National Institute on Drug Abuse. (2018b). *What is heroin and how is it used?* Retrieved from https://www.drugabuse.gov/publications/research-reports/heroin/what-heroin

Nolan, L. J., & Scagnelli, L. M. (2007). Preference for sweet foods and higher body mass index in patients being treated in long-term methadone maintenance. *Substance use & misuse, 42*(10), 1555-1566.

Nosyk, B., Sun, H., Evans, E., Marsh, D. C., Anglin, M. D., Hser, Y. I., & Anis, A. H. (2012). Defining dosing pattern characteristics of successful tapers following methadone maintenance treatment: results from a population-based retrospective cohort study. *Addiction, 107*(9), 1621-1629.

O'Toole, J., Hambly, R., Cox, A., O'Shea, B., & Darker, C. (2014). Methadone-maintained patients in primary care have higher rates of chronic disease and multimorbidity, and use health services more intensively than matched controls. *European Journal of General Practice,20*(4), 275-280. doi:10.3109/13814788.2014.905912

Ouimette, P. E., & Brown, P. J. (2003). *Trauma and substance abuse: Causes, consequences, and treatment of comorbid disorders.* American Psychological Association.

Parks, G. A., & Marlatt, A. (2000). Relapse prevention therapy: A cognitive-behavioral approach. *The National Psychologist, 9*(5), 3.

Patrick, S. W., Schumacher, R. E., Benneyworth, B. D., Krans, E.E., McAllister, J. M., & Davis, M. M. (2012). Neonatal abstinence syndrome and associated health care expenditures: United States, 2000-2009. *JAMA: The Journal of the American Medical Association, 307*(18), 1934–1940.

Pears, K., Capaldi, D. M., & Owen, L. D. (2007). Substance use risk across three generations: the roles of parent discipline practices and inhibitory control. *Psychology of Addictive Behaviors, 21*(3), 373.

Pichini, S., Solimini, R., Berretta, P., Pacifici, R., & Busardò, F. P. (2018). Acute intoxications and fatalities from illicit fentanyl and analogues: an update. *Therapeutic drug monitoring, 40*(1), 38-51.

Prochaska, J. O., & DiClemente, C. C. (1982). Transtheoretical therapy: toward a more integrative model of change. *Psychotherapy: theory, research & practice, 19*(3), 276.

Rajs, J., Petersson, A., Thiblin, I., Olsson-Mortlock, C., Fredriksson, Å., & Eksborg, S. (2004). Nutritional status of deceased illicit drug addicts in Stockholm, Sweden—A longitudinal medicolegal study. *Journal of Forensic Science, 49*(2), 1-10.

Renthal, W., & Nestler, E. J. (2008). Epigenetic mechanisms in drug addiction. *Trends in molecular medicine, 14*(8), 341-350.

Rollnick, S. (2002). Motivational interviewing: Preparing people for change. Guilford Press.

Rosenblum, A., Nuttbrock, L., McQuistion, H., Magura, S., & Joseph, H. (2002). Medical outreach to homeless substance users in New York City: preliminary results. Substance use & misuse, 37(8-10), 1269-1273.

Seal, K. H., Downing, M., Kral, A. H., Singleton-Banks, S., Hammond, J. P., Lorvick, J., ... & Edlin, B. R. (2003). Attitudes about prescribing take-home naloxone to injection drug users for the management of heroin overdose: a survey of street-recruited injectors in the San Francisco Bay Area. *Journal of Urban Health, 80*(2), 291-301.

Seligman, N. S., Salva, N., Hayes, E. J., Dysart, K. C., Pequignot, E. C., & Baxter, J. K. (2008). Predicting length of treatment for neonatal abstinence syndrome in methadone-exposed neonates. *American Journal of Obstetrics and Gynecology, 199*(4), 396.e1-396.e7.

Shapiro, F. (2001). Eye movement desensitization and reprocessing (EMDR): basic principles, protocols, and procedures (2nd ed). The Guilford Press.

Shinderman, M. S., & Maxwell, S. (2000). Sexual dysfunction

associated with methadone maintenance: Treatment with bromocryptine. *Heroin Addiction and Related Clinical Problems, 2,* 9-14.

Siegal, H. A., Li, L., & Rapp, R. C. (2002). Case management as a therapeutic enhancement: Impact on post-treatment criminality. Journal of Addictive Diseases, 21(4), 37-46.

Stern, E. K., & Brenner, D. M. (2018). Spotlight on naldemedine in the treatment of opioid-induced constipation in adult patients with chronic noncancer pain: design, development, and place in therapy. *Journal of pain research, 11,* 195.

Stickgold, R. (2002). EMDR: A putative neurobiological mechanism of action. *Journal of clinical psychology, 58*(1), 61-75.

Strain, E. C., Stitzer, M. L., Liebson, I. A., & Bigelow, G. E. (1993). Dose-response effects of methadone in the treatment of opioid dependence. *Annals of internal medicine, 119*(1), 23-27.

Substance Abuse and Mental Health Services Administration. (2009). *The facts about naltrexone for treatment of opioid addiction* [brochure]. Rockville, MD: JBS International, Inc.

Substance Abuse and Mental Health Services Administration. (2015). *Federal guidelines for opioid treatment programs* [PowerPoint Slides]. Retrieved from http://mpcmh.org/wp-content/uploads/2017/12/SAMHSA_Guidelines_Opiod-Treatment-Programs.pdf

Substance Abuse and Mental Health Services Administration. (2018). *Trauma-informed approach and trauma-specific interventions* Retrieved from https://www.samhsa.gov/nctic/trauma-interventions

Terplan, M., Laird, H. J., Hand, D. J., Wright, T. E., Premkumar, A., Martin, C. E., ... Krans, E. E. (2018). Opioid Detoxification During Pregnancy: A Systematic Review. *Obstetrics and Gynecology, 131*(5), 803–814.

Tuohy, C.M. (2017) Developing an environment of change for the peer recovery support specialist. *Advances in Addiction and Recovery, 5*(3), 5-6.

Umbricht, A., Schroeder, J. R., Antoine, D. G., Tompkins, D. A., Barnhouser, C., Strain, E. C., & Bigelow, G. (2015). Topiramate effect on weight gain during methadone maintenance. *Drug & Alcohol Dependence, 156*, e227.

U.S. Department of Veterans Affairs. (2017a). *PTSD screening instruments.* Retrieved from https://www.ptsd.va.gov/professional/assessment/screens/index.asp

U.S. Department of Veterans Affairs. (2017b). *Treatment of PTSD.* Retrieved from https://www.ptsd.va.gov/public/treatment/therapy-med/treatment-ptsd.asp

U.S. Food & Drug Administration (n.d.). *Labeling & nutrition.* Retrieved from https://www.fda.gov/Food/LabelingNutrition

Velez, M., & Jansson, L. M. (2008). The Opioid dependent mother and newborn dyad: non-pharmacologic care. *Journal of Addiction Medicine, 2*(3), 113–120.

Vocci, F. J., Acri, J., & Elkashef, A. (2005). Medication development for addictive disorders: the state of the science. *American Journal of Psychiatry, 162*(8), 1432-1440.

Wesson, D. R., & Ling, W. (2003). The clinical opiate withdrawal scale (COWS). *Journal of psychoactive drugs, 35*(2), 253-259.

Wilson, K. G., & Murrell, A. R. (2004). Values work in acceptance and commitment therapy. *Mindfulness and acceptance: Expanding the cognitive-behavioral tradition*, 264.

World Health Organization. Department of Mental Health, Substance Abuse, World Health Organization, International Narcotics Control Board, United Nations Office on Drugs, & Crime. (2009). *Guidelines for the psychosocially assisted pharmacological treatment of opioid dependence.* World Health Organization.

Zador, D., Wall, P. M., & Webster, I. (1996). High sugar intake in a group of women on methadone maintenance in South Western Sydney, Australia. *Addiction,91*(7), 1053-1062. doi:10.1046/j.1360-0443.1996.917105311.x

www.ingramcontent.com/pod-product-compliance
Lightning Source LLC
Chambersburg PA
CBHW031422210526
45464CB00005B/2011